# Happier Endings

## A Meditation on Life and Death

## Erica Brown

SIMON & SCHUSTER

NEW YORK   LONDON   TORONTO   SYDNEY   NEW DELHI

Simon & Schuster
1230 Avenue of the Americas
New York, NY 10020

First Simon & Schuster hardcover edition April 2013

SIMON & SCHUSTER and colophon are registered trademarks
of Simon & Schuster, Inc.

For information about special discounts for bulk purchases, please contact Simon &
Schuster Special Sales at 1-866-506-1949 or business@simonandschuster.com.

The Simon & Schuster Speakers Bureau can bring authors to your live event. For more
information or to book an event contact the Simon & Schuster Speakers Bureau at
1-866-248-3049 or visit our website at www.simonspeakers.com.

Designed by Akasha Archer

Manufactured in the United States of America

10   9   8   7   6   5   4   3   2   1

Library of Congress Cataloging-in-Publication Data
   Brown, Erica.
      Happier endings : a meditation on life and death / by Erica Brown.
— 1st Simon & Schuster hardcover ed.
p. cm.
   Includes bibliographical references.
   1. Death—Psychological aspects. I. Title.

BF789.D4B76 2013
128'.5—dc23                    2012018936

ISBN 978-1-4516-4922-2
ISBN 978-1-4516-4924-6 (ebook)

*For Diane*

# Contents

*Preface*
Overcoming the Fear of Death
– 1 –

*Chapter One*
The Business of Death
– 19 –

*Chapter Two*
Pondering the Afterlife
– 49 –

*Chapter Three*
Sanctifying the Body in Death
– 77 –

*Chapter Four*
Death as an Escape
– 117 –

*Chapter Five*
Denial, Resignation, Inspiration
– 149 –

*Chapter Six*
A Different Bucket List
– 177 –

# CONTENTS

*Chapter Seven*
Closing Words
– 211 –

*Chapter Eight*
The Last Apology
– 241 –

*Chapter Nine*
Learning from Grief
– 261 –

*Chapter Ten*
Using Death to Change Your Life
– 289 –

*Epilogue*
– 319 –

*Appendix*
Writing an Ethical Will
– 321 –

*Acknowledgments*
– 329 –

*Notes*
– 331 –

And at last my own death will steal upon me . . .
A gentle, painless death, far from the sea when it comes
To take me down, borne down with the years in ripe old age
With all my people here in blessed peace around me.

—Homer, on the reunion of Penelope and Odysseus

# *Preface*

# Overcoming the Fear of Death

I am afraid to death of death. In my relatively short life, many of my friends, colleagues and students have already passed on, to what I don't know. I've faced the sudden death of others, the suicide of acquaintances, and the slow, tortured end from illness of those I love. Every day I plow through the hours in front of my home computer, at my office or in a supermarket aisle, distracting myself with life's banalities to combat my own subliminal fear of death. I absorb myself in the lives of my children. Intertwining my life with theirs connects me in some irrational way to their youth, pushing the angel of death farther from view. But suddenly—often without noticeable cause—I am ravaged by a primal panic. Everyone dies. I am going to die. The little whisper gets louder. I AM GOING TO DIE.

The escalating noise of this whisper is not odd because death is everywhere, inescapable in its grab for victims. It surrounds us.

According to statisticians, 56 million people die every year. That comes out to 153,000 deaths a day, 107 deaths per minute. The television news barks out death notices in astonishing number, day after day, wearing down our naïve optimism, shocking us with death's randomness. Death shows its face on every newspaper page. There is murder and manslaughter, death by starvation and natural disasters, obituaries of the famous and pictures of suicide bombers stealing the lives of the innocent. Closer to home, friends die of cancer, parents suffer aging, a neighbor loses a child. We wake up trying to quell the existential anguish of it all. We go to a funeral and can't help crying. Sometimes we are crying for ourselves. The death whisper returns: when will it be my turn? And then we go home and make a sandwich, pretending that the drama belongs to someone else. Not us.

Death was a constant shadow in my family's past, a shadow we saw but tried hard to ignore. The fear of it was intense, and over time it jelled into an even more intense stillness and silence. Ignoring death does not make it go away. It made our family woefully underprepared to have the kind of casual frankness with death that makes a person's last imprint one of celebration rather than confusion. I witnessed this close up when my beloved Zeide died. My grandfather died at ninety-five, throwing our family into instant turmoil. He was sick for over a year and in a rehabilitation facility. He was old by any standard except the early chapters of the book of Genesis where characters died at 950. Yet he did not purchase a plot or leave burial instructions. He offered no last words of consolation or wisdom. Out of fear, he did not speak of his death, so no one else did. He was such a monumental figure in my life, yet we never said goodbye.

I was born Jewish to a child survivor of the Holocaust. My mother was born in Poland and spent her young life before the war in Zakrze-wek, a small village south of Lublin. My grandparents sensed danger, left the village and went into hiding. Not long after, all the Jews of

Zakrzewek were rounded up and murdered in one day by the Nazis. My grandparents were concentration camp survivors at Auschwitz, separated from each other and from my mother. My grandfather found my mother in an orphanage in Lublin after his liberation by the Americans, and eventually all three reunited after the war, but not until almost forty members of their—my—family were killed in gas chambers and random shootings. Jewish identity in my childhood home was encapsulated in the faded blue numbers tattooed on my grandparents' arms. Religion was not only something they lived but something they carried: an identity burden, something they couldn't scrub off or get rid of with ease.

I wanted to know what the numbers meant. I spoke with my grandparents about their story and studied the history of the Holocaust. The wholesale death of millions haunted me, not only because the Holocaust is paralyzing in its enormity and travesty but also because I wondered how any survivor could live a normal life. My grandparents moved in the world with grace and laughter. Zeide loved to tell jokes. He was a prankster. But my grandparents, understandably, were superstitious when it came to death. They could and did talk about the tragedy in our family but would never speak of their own deaths. There was something about articulating the language of dying that they believed would precipitate an earlier, untimely death. This fear closed off conversations that needed to happen and emotions that were never properly expressed.

Life can hold more joy but only to a point. It will, one day, be over. Its inevitability should make us fear death less, but instead we fear it more. My grandfather was so choked by its grip that it stymied necessary conversation.

Zeide was no philosopher, mind you. He was a tailor and a dry cleaner, but I wish, between hemming pants, he had read what the French writer Michel de Montaigne once wrote: "To begin depriving death of its greatest advantage over us let us deprive death of its strangeness, let us frequent it, let us get used to it. . . . A man who has learned how to die has unlearned how to be a slave."[1] Learn how to die, unlearn death's strangeness, become its master. It is not death that has a profound stranglehold over us but the fear of death.

That fear is amplified by everything uncertain that death carries with it: the anxious anticipation of not being here, not growing old, not doing what we always wanted to do, not being with those we love, not watching our children grow up and have children of their own. We don't know when we will die, how we will die or how our deaths will affect those around us. But Montaigne was on to something. When we "frequent it" and dissect death's terrors, we find ourselves able to approach our slavish fear of death, invite death into our lives and discuss it, thereby also inviting spiritual growth. We begin to understand, precisely because we cannot live forever, that we have much living and loving to do now. Over time, we can learn to make death our teacher, a teacher of empyrean truths.

For the past several years, I have made death my teacher. In my calmer moments, when the question does not rattle me to the core, I have stepped back and asked myself: is there a better way to die?

Yes there is.

I know this not because I've been blessed with prophecy or an advanced degree in the subject. (Disclaimer: I have not died and come back. That would be an instant bestseller.) I know this because I have been on a personal quest to understand the role that death plays in our lives. My search was jump-started one day in September 2009. On that day, my cousin Alyssa died at age forty. It was unexpected and traumatic. The silence that surrounded death in my family was suddenly broken for the worst possible reason; we were staring at it in front of us with wide, gaping mouths, not knowing what to do or say. I performed my first and only funeral two days later, documented the haunting experience in my journal and decided that it was time to end the family's silence and begin the journey to understanding.

As a Jewish educator for twenty-five years, I needed to understand death not only for myself but for all of those with whom I work closely who also recognize the terror of death and the role it plays in shutting them down and opening them up. I regularly travel with adults through the range of life experiences that percolate major questions and spiritual insights. Confronting the deaths of those we love and facing our own mortality are among the most poignant and frightening steps on life's journey. I began my search with a set of questions, both concrete and abstract. What happens to our bodies after we die? Is there an afterlife? Can an unexpected and sudden death still be beautiful? Does my fear of death contribute in some positive way to my life? In other words, can I leverage the terror and get something out of it? Is there a better way to die, and can we learn it? I wanted to vanquish my fear of death, like some exotic sword-slayer in a medieval thriller, and found an unintended present with my search, the gift of inspiration. I met ordinary people with extraordinary emotional stamina who overcame their fears and left the most important legacy one can leave behind, a better death. Sometimes even a beautiful death.

Studying death exposed me to many different spiritual traditions, philosophical debates, medical practices and cultural beliefs that surround death and the dying. I devoured philosophical and spiritual treatises, ancient mystical texts and psychological and sociological studies. I read numerous books about funeral homes and undertakers-in-training, and I skimmed cemetery and hospice manuals. I learned about the chemistry of cremation, the intricacies of Japanese burial ceremonies and even performed a ritual bath on a dead woman. Most importantly, I interviewed dozens of remarkable people who made themselves vulnerable through our conversations about the most fragile of human experiences, many of them in tears as we spoke.

Here's some of what I learned: the grim reaper is not always grim; our last days *can* be the most loving time of life; last words have remarkable staying power; and learning about the mechanics of how we *do* death can make the prospect less daunting. The more prepared we are for the logistics of death, the less those who profit from death (the so-called death industry) can exploit us. The more open we are about our own deaths, the more prepared our survivors will be to face their own ultimate truths one day. The more emotionally generous we are with words, affection and regrets, the easier it will be to control the fear. We *can* achieve happier endings.

Studying death through speaking to the dying and their survivors also made me question Elisabeth Kübler-Ross, the physician and writer, whose five stages of grief radically altered the way we think about death and loss. Denial, anger, bargaining, depression and acceptance have become such an axiomatic understanding of loss that we may, as a result, limit our fullest and most warming experience of death. I am no longer convinced that these stages truly capture what is taking place during the period when one's death or the death of someone we love is imminent. Many therapists have questioned Kübler-Ross's stages, believing that the word "stage" may be misleading. Not everyone experiences all five stages, nor do these stages occur in a linear fashion, with people waiting for one stage to stop and the next to begin. My problem with this ladder of loss is that it is missing its most important rung. The last, most potent stage or development within the framework of loss is not acceptance. It is inspiration. I humbly believe Kübler-Ross missed something in her categorization that may be the key to the fine art of dying well, if we can ever truly call it that.

I turned Kübler-Ross's list into a different and abbreviated outline in my own mind. Denial is undoubtedly the first stage, bold and tenacious. Then, in my new death outline, anger, bargaining and depression become subsumed under denial as different manifestations of the unwillingness to accept death. They are all—anger, bargaining and depression—mechanisms of denial. They represent different fields of the battleground, the fight against a truth that cannot be broken. Kübler-Ross's acceptance turned into resignation in my new scheme. There is a moment when the fight ends and the resignation begins.

"Acceptance" is a little too positive to describe this stage. It gives the impression of being welcome, and death is rarely welcome. If we define "acceptance" as consent or receiving something with approval or favor, then "acceptance" becomes too cheery for what most who grieve experience. "Resignation" seems the semantically more appropriate word. We submit to the inevitability of our fate, aggressively, passively or unresistingly. We tell ourselves: This is real. It will not go away. It is a new fact of our existence, which is one of the only old facts of human existence. In happier endings, the observation "This is real" is twinned with the maturing understanding "I am unprepared." And this confession is critical to achieving the next stage: "I *need* to be prepared."

Once someone is able to utter these words—"I need to be prepared"—a flood of change takes place that enables us to face death without fear. This is the stage I call "inspiration," a stage that never appeared in Kübler-Ross's framework but appeared in virtually every conversation I had with a person or family who managed to do death better. The intentional decision to become better prepared for death gives the dying permission to love more fully, to say the words they've wanted to say for a lifetime, to repair and heal troubled relationships, and to entertain a range of ethereal and spiritual thoughts and actions often previously closed off, sealed or masked by the pragmata of everyday anxieties. It gives the family the chance to reach out to the dying with an emotional range previously unknown or unexperienced. By not acknowledging that the stage of inspiration exists, many never believe that it is possible; they retain the stubborn belief that acceptance alone is the last station. In so doing, they deny themselves the beautiful closure that only the enlightened ever achieve but that is a possibility for almost everyone.

A successful businessman in his fifties mourned the fact that no one was able to say "Dad's dying" after three stressful weeks in the hospital and three additional weeks at home. "It happened so fast," his son lamented to me one morning over coffee. Stuck in the quicksand of denial, the family did not realize that when a nurse wheeled Dad out to a family dinner and he addressed his wife and each son that he was actually saying goodbye. How tender that dinner could have been had they opened their eyes and seen what was really going on. "He was saying goodbye, and none of us realized until long after it happened." Inspiration is not a stage of grief. It is an admission of possibility. It is the last gift we give the living.

My exploration of death began with questions I thought had no answers. It ended—as much as any such journey can ever end—with answers that were personally transformative. And because I know that you find this hard to believe, I have to introduce you to my teachers, each of whom is worth a thousand books on death. Good teachers are those who die well and show us how with their very lives. My teachers dot the pages that follow. First let me introduce you to Rose. Rose was Connie's mother.


Not long after her mother died, Connie and I met on a sparkling San Francisco afternoon outside the museum she once directed. She took me on a tour, and toward the end of our walk, we spoke about her mother.

"I'm so sorry to hear about her death," I said, expressing my deepest condolences.

Connie beamed. "Don't be sorry. My mother had the most beautiful death."

*That's odd*, I thought. Such a response in the face of consolation was quite rare. *There must be a story here.* Connie told me that in a month she was going on a trip with her four sisters to spread her mother's ashes on a ski slope. There was a lot to say, and she would tell me all about it when she got back.

Rosemarie—or Rose, as she was called—died in her early eighties in Idaho. She had lupus for thirty years and eventually died of related complications. Connie swore you'd never know about her mother's chronic condition because her mother made it a practice not to complain about being ill. Rose lived her life full of spirit, and she also died that way.

I wondered what it meant to die full of spirit. Connie explained. Rose's husband, Connie's father, had committed suicide when Connie was only fifteen; both of Rose's parents died before she was ten, leaving her an orphan. Rose was on intimate terms with death. Suffering was the measure of her life. Rose wanted to undo this upbringing of pain in raising her own five daughters. There must be a better way to do death, she reckoned. So Rose talked about death casually and often, to the point where the family joke involved the neighborhood funeral home, Metcalf's.

"So, Mother, when are you going to Metcalf's?"

"Is it time to go to Metcalf's?"

Rose had a host of illnesses. As she aged into more severe pain, Rose was told that she would have to undergo dialysis. She had always had a very close relationship with her doctors; Rose knew her options and was not in denial about what lay ahead. Rose did not want the hospital life associated with dialysis and decided instead to soldier through her pain until the end. Connie told me about an incident, which happened several months in advance of Rose's death, that most illustrated her mother's attitude toward her health. Rose had traveled from Idaho each month to see a world specialist in San Francisco as her condition worsened. The doctor casually asked her if anything had happened to her in the intervening month, and Rose said that nothing unusual had occurred. "What do you mean, Mother?" Connie interrupted forcefully. "Did you forget that you were diagnosed with breast cancer since we were last here?"

Rose had not forgotten about the cancer. She just would not let it get in her way. She pushed it away with dignity. In her view, every day presented another chance to live, so why should she dwell on dying? She was not going to carry her cancer around, lugging it about like a heavy suitcase, a conversation-stopper. She was determined that sickness would neither define nor limit her. Rose knew herself well enough to know that she needed to retain control of the decision-making that so often imperceptibly slips through the fingers of the dying. To that end, years before sickness ate away at her, Rose held what Connie called a tag sale in her house. She told the girls to label everything in the house they wanted and explained which sister would be the executor of her will and why. She divided up the better jewelry and organized her papers and set out her burial wishes. In Connie's words:

It was the best gift she gave us. Nothing made my mother happier than when we were all around her and all got along. She made all these plans not because she was a controlling person but because she didn't want us to fight about what she left. She saw too many families broken apart because of fighting over an inheritance and she wanted us to know what she wanted. None of us was going to second-guess what she wanted, as so many people do. And that was her last and best gift because it worked.

What Connie described touched a deep emotional chord with me. Having gone through too many death scenes where I watched families torn apart by financial issues that really amounted to sibling rivalry and envy—arguing over small items or certain that a parent or a spouse wanted to be buried one way and not another—it became obvious that survivors don't want to betray the desires of the deceased but often have no idea what those desires are. When survivors are left to second-guess, every possibility spells out unhappiness in a different way, and the living suffer the displeasure more than the dead. Rose prepared her family because she did not want her death to be a source of family infighting.

For months, Connie and her sisters took turns staying beside their mother. Connie never minded cleaning and bathing Rose or changing her clothing and taking her to the bathroom. She thought it was moving to tend to her mother's most basic needs. When Rose protested, Connie replied that Rose had done all of this and more when she was a baby, and it was Connie's turn now. "She said she didn't want me to see her this way, but I think she was really touched that we took care of her." Connie made me realize that the most salient reason we don't take care of those who are dying may be to protect ourselves from the reality of our own deaths. It's not fair to the dying. They need us, and we are not there because we do not want to look in that mirror. They need us to have more courage than that. Connie could take care of her mother because her mother taught her not to be afraid of death.

One of Connie's cousins who believed in contacting spirits in the afterlife set her up with a spirit reader about a month after Rose passed away. The woman knew nothing about Connie's life or Rose's death, but she told her that her mother thanked her for taking care of her at the end. This reassured Connie that Rose's dignity had not been compromised. Then, with a laugh, Connie brushed off the spirit reader.

She went back for a second visit, and everything the spirit reader said was just plain wrong. "But that first message, it really sounded like something my mom would say."

Rose was a stickler in the personal care department. The sisters knew the end was near when Rose came home from her final visit to the hospital and scheduled and then canceled a manicure and an in-home hairdressing appointment for the next day. Rose told Connie that she was just wasn't up to it.

"That's when I knew," Connie said.


Connie described with great tenderness the moment her mother died. Mike, Rose's second husband of thirty-five years, insisted on being with Rose constantly. The day of the canceled appointments, Mike went to take a shower while Connie hovered near her mother. Rose lay on the couch sleeping. "Suddenly her breathing changed dramatically, and I screamed out for Mike. We were both there the moment she passed away. It was incredible." The family was already en route, and when one of her other sisters arrived, the three of them moved the body to Rose's own bed. Connie's voice lowered slightly when she shared what this moment was like for her.

My mother weighed so little in those last weeks. She had also lost inches of her height over the years. We each positioned ourselves to move her, and I was responsible for holding up her middle. She was probably four foot eight and not even ninety pounds, but when we moved her, she was so heavy, so very heavy. And that's when I knew that her spirit left her. Her spirit made her light, and when her spirit left, her body was just so unexpectedly heavy. I remember thinking that.

Soon, all the family had gathered around Rose in her bedroom. They sat on the bed, all of the sisters together, and told stories about their mother. They even put lipstick on Rose because that was what they felt she would have done in front of her girls. Connie recalled that little flourish with fondness and then described what it meant to have everyone together: "It was what she would have wanted, what she most loved: her girls all around her, talking with each other and just being together."

Rose left very specific burial instructions and nothing to chance. She wanted her body to be cremated, and she wanted Mike and each of the girls to take a packet of her ashes and throw them on a ski slope in Sun Valley, Idaho. She was even specific about the slope. "My mother was a great skier, and she skied even when her bones were brittle and always breaking. We just could not get that crazy woman to stop. She wanted us to spread her ashes over one run, Christian's Gold. And she wanted that run and not any other because she didn't like all the slopes."

The night before going to the ski slope, the sisters held a dinner party for about twenty of Rose's close friends. They toasted her and celebrated her life through stories. They praised Rose for creating real closure with her friends and with Mike. Months after Rose's death, Mike called Connie to ask her to repeat a conversation between Rose and Mike that Connie had witnessed. "Connie, did Rose really say that there should be another Mrs. Fishman? Did you really hear that?" Mike wanted to make sure he understood Rose correctly. She wanted life to go on for everyone. She wanted Mike to have as much love without her as they knew together in their marriage—none of the cessation W. H. Auden depicts in "Funeral Blues" where all the clocks are asked to stop, where time itself pauses in the face of loss. Life would go on. Life must go on. Rose demanded that it should.

Connie wondered how the dispersal of ashes was going to work. She also was not sure it was legal. I was pretty curious myself. I had certainly heard of people who wanted to be cremated and buried at sea. And I knew of someone whose ashes were stuffed into a champagne bottle at a military funeral. Yet for all the odd stories I collected over the years, I never heard of someone who loved skiing so much that she wanted to spend her eternal life on a ski slope. It seemed a little cold for my taste.

Connie explained that her mother hated cemeteries. Because Rose had lost her parents so young, visiting gravesites probably was an onerous and regular part of Rose's young life. Maybe she didn't want that memory for her daughters or maybe she just didn't want that kind of eternal company. Cemeteries are lonely and quiet, flat and eerie. Rose had a point. Why not "live" among happy people having fun in a gorgeous place with an expansive view where death seems so far away?

While Connie did not have trouble coming to terms with her mother's last request, she was stuck on the logistics. "I mean, really, how were we going to divide up her ashes and get them in a few different pouches? I just couldn't figure it out." But this detail, in the end, was not complicated. The funeral home that cremated Rose placed the ashes in individual white pouches, and Mike distributed them to each of the girls and took one for himself. Connie described the scene with a note of bemusement: "So there we were in the car, driving to the mountain in our ski gear and our boots, and we each had a piece of my mother with us. It was just so very odd. And again, her ashes felt really, really heavy. I guess I expected them to be light."

It was a cold, sunny day when they set out for the mountaintop, just the kind of day that was perfect for skiing, even—apparently—if you were no longer alive. Up on the top of the slope, they each interpreted Rose's last wish differently. One sister went to the side of the slope and placed the ashes in the crux of a tree. One put them nearer to the bottom so that Rose could metaphorically finish the run. Another felt that her mother's ashes should be on the top of the slope looking down in anticipation of the run. Connie skied over to a clump of trees and scattered the ashes into the wind and the trees. Another sister spread them out as she slowly skied down the trail. This last choice had some unintended consequences for Connie:

> As I was skiing down the mountain having thrown out my mother's ashes, I realized that I was actually skiing on my mother's ashes because now I knew what they looked like. They were the ashes my sister let go of on the slope. For a minute I thought, *I am actually skiing on my mother.*

Connie paused, understanding that this strange coincidence was unusual by any standards, and then added, "It felt great. Really great." She and the family had honored her mother's last request in every detail. It offered potent solace.

> When we all got to the bottom and exchanged stories about where we put our ashes and what we felt, we all shared the same exact feeling: a huge weight had been lifted. We had done exactly what she wanted. And I knew that once her physical body was no longer with us in any way, that her spirit was there, all spirit. And it's with me every day. It's with me now. I talk to her all the time . . .

What Connie was describing was not the absence of her mother but the enduring gift of her mother's presence.

It was then that I realized—with the clarity that comes when an abstract idea manifests itself concretely—that in my quest for a better death, people really could have a happier ending, a beautiful death, despite illness, despite suffering, even with incalculable losses. Rose had vanquished her fear and taught her daughters not to be afraid of death, and now she was teaching me as well. Death is life's only certainty, and death was going to come. Rose knew it, so why deny it? Rose talked openly about it with her doctors and her family, made tough decisions about it and spelled out all requests related to it in detail. She divided up her material possessions and gave them away in her lifetime because she didn't want her death to be associated with arguments, resentment or envy. She generously gave permission for others to continue without her. She said whatever she needed to say. She spent her last days eating French fries and ice cream instead of hooked up to dialysis. She taught her daughters to embrace death so that they could live fully.

Ultimately, Rose gave her family a happy ending because she was able to confront her death without fear. In Connie's words, "Losing her body made me understand how much she will always live within me. Always." If Rose's soul lives on in Connie, then Rose only died in one sense of the word. Her ending was, in some of the most critical ways, not an ending at all. Connie still holds her mother close.

Rose also taught me that a happier ending has two vantage points: the first from the person who is dying and the second from those left behind. Learning how to overcome the fear of death requires moving in and out of these viewpoints almost seamlessly. The dying who overcome fear learn to die better, and those who watch them die learn to die better as well.

Thank you, Rose. I didn't really believe in a beautiful death until Connie introduced us. Thank you for becoming a student of death so that you could become my teacher.


In the late summer of 1827, the Hasidic master Rabbi Simcha Bunim of Przysucha was ailing and close to death. His wife stood beside him, awash in bitter tears. Finally, he turned to her in irritation and demanded silence. Rabbi Bunim could not understand why his wife was crying, waiting as he had for this moment. With one sentence he explained: "My whole life was only that I should learn to die."

*Chapter One*

# The Business of Death

Aunt Diane and Uncle Roy found Alyssa's body collapsed on the floor in her apartment late one Wednesday afternoon in September after no one had answered her phone for many hours. That afternoon, everything about their lives changed forever. It was every parent's nightmare stretched out before them in graphic horror. In her memoir *The Year of Magical Thinking,* Joan Didion sums up those painful minutes of devastation that transform families when her own husband died suddenly of a heart attack in the living room: "Life changes fast. Life changes in the instant. You sit down to dinner and life as you know it ends."

Alyssa had also died alone, reflecting one of our most persistent fears. We are terrified to die by ourselves, left alone and undiscovered for a long time. The Japanese have a word for it: *kodokushi.* Translated loosely, it means "lonely death." In *Psychology Today,* Professor Bella

DePaulo contends that this fear is often treated as a threat among singles but questions its validity as a reason to couple up. The likelihood of dying alone is not minimized by marriage necessarily, argues E. Kay Trimberger, author of *The New Single Woman*, but by whether or not you have an active and loving circle of friends.[1] Yet we understand this often unarticulated anxiety; to die alone seems to symbolize in the most ultimate sense the anomie of an empty society.[2] There will be no one to hear the last word that we ever say, no one to hold a hand and no one to see the last breath imperceptibly leave us.

I once went out for coffee with an older man in one of my classes who had lost his wife a few years back and was clearly not over the pain. "I'm lonely. I don't want to spend my last years alone. I don't want to die alone." He told me that the pain of his wife's absence was so profound that he slept at night with a pile of books in his bed in the place his wife had occupied for the dozens of years they were married. He loved her. He loved books. He thought that perhaps there was some transference of these loves that would bring him a modicum of solace. If books were at his side when he died, he would not have to die alone.

Diane and Roy did not suspect foul play or that Alyssa had taken her own life. They had—and still have—no idea what really happened. Alyssa struggled mightily in her life with her own demons. As a teenager, she went through a period of months when she was afraid to leave the house, and she struggled with other phobias, even as she fought her parents for independence. She never finished her education in the classic sense, but after a string of jobs, she studied to be a nurse's assistant and stabilized her employment. She was married for a brief and rough few months. It was a beautiful wedding. In her white dress and with her wide smile, it seemed that she had finally figured herself out. But the fairy-tale picture of wedding happiness soon gave way to a harsher reality. Not long after her separation, she joined her parents in Florida and moved into her own apartment a few miles away. Alyssa was needy but very big-hearted. She loved her dog, Elle, and her niece and nephew, and she wanted a happy family like the ones she saw on TV screens and in magazines. She desperately wanted to be a mother.

Within an hour of finding her, Diane and Roy were surrounded by police officers. My aunt called me screaming. When I got her, between sobs, to tell me what happened, she said only two words and then released another anguished cry: "She's dead." She and Roy had lost their only daughter.

Alyssa's body was placed in a thick plastic bag on a rolling stretcher. Diane needed a prayer. "What should I say before they take her away?" she said in a whisper. I listed some prayers in Hebrew that are typically recited. "I don't know any of that Hebrew. You say something," and she put the phone on the body bag. I recited a few psalms and the central prayer of Judaism, the Shema. I told her that she and my uncle should ask *mechila*, "forgiveness," from Alyssa. In Jewish tradition, emotional closure is critical and tightly ritualized, and it involves atonement. We ask forgiveness of the dead, and for some people this is the hardest and starkest reality of saying farewell. That last "I'm sorry for everything" is both a letting go and a reminder that whatever difficulties and arguments may have characterized the relationship between the living and the dead, all must be forgiven. There are no more chances for reconciliation or for the conversation you meant to have but never did.

When a body is placed in a bag, or on a stretcher or in a casket, an unnerving change happens to our perceptions of existence. We realize the stark and unambiguous reality that something as large as life can be contained in an incredibly small space. Professor James Kugel in his book *In the Valley of the Shadow*—ruminations on the foundations of religion into which he weaves his personal trial with cancer—writes that he is always "astonished by the smallness of the freshly dug, open holes you see here and there in the cemetery grounds. *Can a whole human being fit in there, a whole human life?* Yes. No problem."[3]

We can—each of us—be contained in a small spit of earth. The hole reduces all of human life to a dark, containable, insignificant space. I lingered on Kugel's words, "a whole human life," having just had the same thought when a beloved friend, a pediatric oncologist, died of cancer himself. He was a larger-than-life sort of fellow. He loved to eat and talk and teach. He was exuberant. And so, in some wrong irony of the universe, he got thyroid cancer and could not eat and could not talk and could not teach. And then I saw the hole they dug at the cemetery to bury him. Could it possibly contain him? It did. When he was fifty-one, cancer had made him smaller and smaller, and he shrunk right out of his life, two weeks before becoming a grandfather. Gone. I remember a light rain mixed with the afternoon sun right after the burial. A rainbow spread across the cemetery. One of his children said, "That was just the sort of thing that Dad would have planned." He was a colorful person who seemed to have choreographed his own end. A rainbow was perfect. It just made sense.

I understood from the shakiness in Diane's voice that she and Roy could not be alone, so I promised to be there soon and booked a one-way ticket. From a distance, my husband and I made calls to morgues, the police station, detectives, and the pathologist's office to try to understand what had happened and when the body would be released. We wanted to spare Diane and Roy the anguish of these conversations. They had enough pain to manage. I tried desperately to secure a rabbi to visit the home, and, through an internet search and various connections, someone showed up late that evening. Suddenly the need for rituals was profound, but it's hard to conjure up a spiritual cushion quickly. Religious communities have a way of stepping in to do death, directing us and pushing us forward into the abyss of pain with a safety net of company and highly choreographed behaviors. Death rituals in all faiths are small, meaningful acts of emotional closure that are attempted but never guaranteed. But Diane and Roy were not part of a faith community. Jews bury the dead as close to the time of death as possible. We tried to have Alyssa's body released in a timely way. Like so many people unprepared for death, they did not know what to do. The next twenty-four hours were a surreal slap of American death, an unimaginable walk through a really bad movie. It was the very opposite of a good death. It came with price tags and quick, uncomfortable decisions that were permanent, with virtually no time to think and made in the dense, emotional fog of loss.

I only fully understood that death is often accompanied by a slick-haired salesman when Alyssa died. Death is big business. The average amount spent on a funeral today ranges between $5,000 and $10,000. An estate lawyer I know told me that the family of one of his deceased clients spent $45,000 on his funeral, $19,000 of it on an elaborate mausoleum. "It's what they needed to do. It seems like things weren't going so well for them as a family." Guilt over a bad relationship can be costly, and no one knows how to exploit that guilt better than some funeral home directors.

Although no one can put a price on a life, death does have a price. Jessica Mitford, whose revolutionary book *The American Way of Death* questioned just about every assumption we have about the way we were "doing death" in America, was outraged by the price of dying. Her husband, a labor lawyer, was angry about exploitation in the funeral industry and got his wife, a writer, fired up about it. Mitford bought a pile of trade magazines and carefully read the articles and the ads, discovering a world of sales she never knew existed. One ad said that keeping up with the Joneses was not only about the high status of living but the high status of dying. Other ads appealed to the search for excellence. Why settle for anything less than the craftsmanship, beauty, comfort and durability you expect in a living room set when it comes to your casket?

Appalled by these sentiments and others, Mitford wrote a magazine article to out these practices, only to find that every major trade magazine rejected it. It finally found a home in a small publication and, when a progressive funeral society ordered 10,000 reprints, her ideas sailed fast and furiously into the fighting fever of the 1960s. A movement was born, and Mitford became its poster child. The book that emerged quickly changed funeral practices. Clients were suddenly more suspicious of what they were being sold and why. Clergy felt relief that someone was finally exposing dishonest business practices that now had ritual and myth attached to them. The notion that people needed a "memory picture"—a view of the deceased made-up and embalmed—because it was important for closure was finally being questioned. So was the "grief therapy" that was (and still is) regularly offered as a service in many funeral homes. The undertaker was moving into a therapist role but with few of the requisite qualifications. Sanitizing or denying the reality of death in the way that the dead are buried often prolongs and attenuates emotional turmoil. It's hard for an undertaker to be a grief therapist because by dolling up the dead, he or she may actually be getting in the way of confronting the reality of death.

People who are grieving and simply cannot think clearly are perfect targets for unethical practices. They rush into decisions. They are heavily influenced by what they see in front of them and don't want money to get in the way of their grief. Where people spending several thousand dollars might normally shop around, funeral homes tend to be a first-stop-only store for burial. You take what's on offer because you don't know any better and are limited to what is placed before you. And bargain shoppers take note: there are no sales.

Mitford describes in detail the casket walk that is presented by funeral directors in their showrooms. Caskets in different price ranges are strategically placed, and the tour of the casket room often moves in a triangle formation so that by the time the shopper is done, he or she has moved out of one price range and into another. You shouldn't bury old Uncle Fred in the cheapest casket, and after the guilt walk you won't. Most people go for the midrange casket because they don't want to seem ostentatious in their choices, but neither do they want to be the family cheapskates. That's exactly what the walk is designed to do: price you above your original intentions. This reminds me of a cartoon where a man in a suit escorts a couple into a casket room and says, "What will it take to put one of you into a brand new Eterna 5000 today?"[4] If buying a casket feels like buying a car, it is because it *is* like buying a car. And close to the same price of a used one. Unfortunately, there doesn't seem to be much of a market for used caskets.

Early the next afternoon, I arrived at Diane and Roy's house in Florida. My grandmother, aunt, uncle, cousin and his wife were all sitting on the brown leather couches in the family room in a stupor. A rabbi was arguing with them about how to bury Alyssa. My aunt suspected that Alyssa would have been scared to be buried in the ground, having once said as much. Because of the water tables in Florida, many people are buried aboveground in vaults, but a traditional Jewish funeral requires burial in the earth. In the words of the book of Job, we go back to the earth that we come from. In Hebrew, the name Adam, the first primordial being, comes from the word *adama*, "earth." Nothing can be more natural. We let the body go back to where it belongs, in Mother Earth. The rabbi would not perform the ceremony if the family picked a vault burial, but he lacked the sensitivity to help them understand the spiritual message behind these choices. I asked him politely to leave, and I drove my aunt and uncle to the Eternal Light Memorial Gardens cemetery. To make the decision, they needed to see the options and make them real.

In what felt like thousand-degree heat, we walked to the various available plot sites and began the heart-wrenching decision of where Alyssa should lie eternally. Diane was crying, her whole body trembling continuously; she said she didn't care. And she didn't at that moment, because it was simply too overwhelming to bury your daughter and to be in this mall of death wares, where a man in a bad toupee and a polyester suit was selling waterfront plots for more, gravestones near a mausoleum for less. There was no room and no time for buyer's remorse.

Diane's first shrug of not caring where Alyssa would be buried soon gave way to caring a great deal. They decided to bury Alyssa in the ground. Diane looked for mystical signs to give her direction in burying her child somewhere that signified some small part of Alyssa's life. A butterfly flitting—maybe that was the spot. The shade of a leafy tree: Alyssa would have liked that. We tried to ignore the bugs and heat as we walked from place to place. Diane and Roy were afraid for Alyssa to be alone. She had suffered enough loneliness for one lifetime. I asked my aunt and uncle where they planned to be buried, but they had not decided that yet, until that Thursday. "Maybe you want to be buried next to her so she won't be alone?" I suggested. We looked for a site for three. It got more complicated to locate a plot for three, but it eased the edge of fear just a bit.

You can't be buried just anywhere in a cemetery. Some patches are filled and crowded. New spaces have to be filled systematically. Diane wasn't happy with the new burial area, but she didn't have much choice if she wanted a three-plot site. Roy noiselessly followed her lead. She walked back and forth and then lay down on the ground to see if this was where she too would place eternal roots. "Okay. This is okay. We'll take this," she told our salesperson. Thinking that she came to bury one person, she left that day with three plots. "Do you want the $4,000 marble bench with her name on it for visitation?" said the real estate agent of death, implying that any committed visitor would, of course, opt for it. "No." Diane was done.

Mosquitoes swarmed the grass, and I kept swiping them from my ankles, aware of the small irritations in the face of life's much larger irritations. As we walked, Diane asked questions with urgency.

"What will happen to her soul?"

"I don't know. Nobody knows, Diane."

"What does Judaism say?"

"Judaism says lots of different things, but there's no one answer."

Bad answer. I felt foolish saying this, and I knew as it left my mouth how unsatisfactory it sounded. Yet that's what happens when you have a four-thousand-year-old tradition of debate. There is no one answer. No one has died and come back to tell us. Maimonides, the medieval philosopher and physician, says that when we work on our spiritual lives in this world, our souls will live on in another, free of the body, as our bodies go back to the earth. The body holds the soul, but if we don't spend time developing and nurturing the soul, then when the body dies, there is no soul to live beyond its physical casing. I did not tell this to Diane. Words escaped me. She did not want to know about Maimonides at that moment. Every question was really a restatement of one word: why. And for that, there were no satisfactory answers. We were quiet for a while as we thought about Alyssa's soul.

Then we drove to the funeral home to arrange for the burial the next day. Diane was lying across the backseat of the car, quivering with tears. Who drives to a funeral home to bury a child? "Why? Why?" The same question tumbled out again and again. Roy and I said nothing.

We were ushered into an office and sat nervously waiting for the funeral director, who came in suited and somber and extended an arm in handshake and consolation. He had the practiced sad voice of a death professional as he handed me some papers with a list of services. Diane grimly checked the boxes. There was the refrigeration fee, the morgue fee, the *tahara* (ritual purification), the hairstyling (if necessary), the *shemira* services, where a person stays up all night with the body reciting psalms, the shroud costs. There was the cost of the casket. Diane looked to the funeral director for guidance and compassion, but the dark wood desk starkly separated those who were grieving from those who were working.

The casket room was down the hall; it was also the room that held Alyssa's body, so I only peeked through the doorway. It was time for the casket walk. All the caskets were named after biblical heroes. The Asher casket was more expensive than the Esther model. Asher was made of burled wood with a silk lining; Esther was just a simple maple. There was also the Abraham, the Joshua and the Daniel; biblical patriarchs and matriarchs graced life's end as retail objects with names like women's shoes or wigs. There was also a magazine-like rack of side panels in the corner that could be placed, for an additional fee, on the sides of the casket, like car accessories. If you were a military person you could have a casket sporting a flag; others might want one with a flower theme or a watercolored landscape of a sailboat on the sea. While I did not see any Major League Baseball caskets in this Jewish funeral home, I had seen pictures elsewhere. I knew that you could go down with your team, even if they were doing well that season. There were no prices for the caskets. You had to ask. I was astonished at the lineup and followed up later when I was home with an online price-check.

Costco, as it turns out, has a line of cheaper caskets, but none have the same Old Testament names. Instead, you can get the Edward, the Continental, or the Kentucky Rose. If I were Christian it would have been a toss-up between the In God's Care line and The Lady of Guadalupe casket. I like any interior that features a little pillow. It's more comforting somehow. Other attractive features of my Lady include:

- ice-blue crepe interior
- embroidered Lady of Guadalupe head panel
- gold-colored handles with Lady of Guadalupe appliqués
- adjustable bed and mattress

The last feature is particularly important to me because I'm not a great sleeper. I wasn't sure I loved the ice-blue interior color. Personally, it's a little frosty, and although Costco does note that they "have selected the most popular styles and colors, with the highest quality linings," they currently do not offer color choices. It is a limiting factor.

I was also intrigued by a comment made to a journalist who did some research into casket sales. When he inquired about the difference between caskets for men and women, he was told by one funeral director that "ladies' caskets are more tapered with chamfered edges, therefore considered more 'slimming.'"[5] I will certainly be pursuing that option: I am not going to be buried in a fat casket. No way.

It's hard enough to get to a discount warehouse on an ordinary day, but at times of emotional stress it's worse. They don't carry multiple styles in every store either. I recommend online ordering even with the unpredictability of shipping times. Costco does offer expedited shipping on caskets, and the Federal Trade Commission requires funeral homes to accept any casket purchased from an outside source although they recommend that the purchaser notify the funeral home of their purchase within one business day. I guess it must be like walking into a bookstore and then buying the book on Amazon instead. It's a real bummer for the funeral home.

What about the return policy? Costco will only accept the return of a casket due to freight or cosmetic damage from shipping. Basically, you're stuck with it. So if you're thinking of picking out your eternal, cushioned closet and you'd never go retail, make sure you pick a classic style that can weather fashion changes.

If you don't like anything at Costco, you can try BestPriceCasket .com. As they say on their home page: "We supply funeral homes and we also sell directly to you! Same Price. Buy Direct." It's a compelling pitch, and it's even more convincing when you see their online advice bold and underlined: "Do Not Tell The Funeral Home About Purchasing Our Casket Before You Get Their Itemized Funeral Price List. Call Us Before Talking to ANY Funeral Home, Because Everything You Tell the Funeral Home Affects Your Funeral Pricing. We Will Tell You What to Say."

Clearly they know something that we don't. I wanted to know their trade secret, so I called.

"Best Price. Can I help you?"

"I want to know what to say to a funeral home if I order a casket from you."

"Let me put you through to sales."

I waited for a long time on hold (but not an eternity!), since I could save thousands—and if we're talking about an eternity then a few more minutes wouldn't really matter. When a saleswoman did pick up, I repeated the question and listened to her answer.

"Ask for an itemized price list and then compare prices. It's like a car dealership. You don't go in there acting like you've got a lot of money. Get the best price while obviously getting what you think your loved one wants. A lot of them [funeral homes] are used to it by now because there are a lot of online dealers. They're losing money. If you get an itemized price list, they can't try to compensate for the loss of the casket fee. They can't overcharge you at that point." In other words, if you do tell a funeral home up front that you're buying a casket elsewhere, they may try to make up the difference in other associated burial fees. The itemized list is the key. The woman in sales closed her presentation with an acknowledgment of the difficulty: "If you've never dealt with it, it can be a really high-pressure sale."

She asked me where I was from and said that they ship to my local airport once a week. "We ship all over the United States. It's no problem getting a casket to you within a day."

I think I'll wait.


While we sat in the funeral director's office, Diane looked at me with confusion. Most of the other services were basic and required. Alyssa would have no hairstyling, but the morgue fee was nonnegotiable. The list of check marks on the bill, line items of hell, increased. *It's only money,* I thought—but it's also money. You never want to feel like you skinflinted your nearest and dearest because you didn't buy her the burled wood. My husband, as a medical resident, once stumbled on the newspaper obituary of a patient who had died in the emergency room (not my husband's fault). The man's son had written: "And I know that wherever my father is right now, he got there cheaper than anyone else." I guess he didn't go for the burled wood either.

Traditionally Jews are buried in simple pine caskets. The Talmud decreed over two thousand years ago that all Jews are to be buried in the same type of shroud and the same type of casket. We are all departing the same world, and we have to leave in the same way. Death is the great economic equalizer in Jewish law. Whatever death accessories were displayed on the shelves that day were a leftover from someone else's tradition. My uncle was relieved about the simple option and remembered that he had learned somewhere that Jews leave this world simply. The casket was of yellow pine with a simple Star of David on the top center panel. Later, when we stood by the casket as it was rolled from the hearse to her burial spot, I meditated on that star, holding on to that last image I would associate with my cousin.

Audrey Gordon, who was once an assistant to Kübler-Ross, wonders in her writings about the rationale behind excessive casket purchases, suggesting that the "expense is often the way that a family represses its guilt over past treatment of the dead or defends itself against its feelings of anger because the loved one has abandoned them. These feelings need to be worked through as a normal part of the process of grief so that later memories of the deceased can be enjoyed without pain or avoidance."[6]

Gordon unearths the often unhealthy subterranean tensions that travel in families around burial practices that, ironically, bury the problems more than they bury the dead. The New Yorker recently carried a cartoon of a middle-aged woman in black standing before a lectern. Behind her was an elevated casket. She addressed the guests at the funeral: "Mother wouldn't have wanted us to feel sad—she'd want us to feel guilty."[7]

After Diane and Roy wrote out a few checks, the funeral director asked if they would like to see Alyssa and say goodbye to her. My aunt asked if I would join them, but I wanted to give them the privacy of their last farewell. I had not found her lying dead on the floor, and I wanted to keep one memory picture clear in my head. It was not the Alyssa the last time I saw her but my first cousin at age six or seven. She is in a photograph at her ballet-school production, wearing a sky-blue tutu and an ornate bonnet. Against a white studio background, she bends forward like a blue flower with one of her feet pointing upward. She has a big smile, very sure of herself for the audience. Later, when my aunt and I sorted out photos of Alyssa to put out on the coffee table for the *shiva*, we saw that big smile again: a still-life in heels at her high-school prom, a serious third-grader holding an open notebook, a breathing, laughing, birthday-party-going kid. "We loved making birthday parties," Diane said with a sigh. I brought the pictures downstairs and put them all over the coffee table. At a *shiva* people are supposed to talk about the dead, not about the mundane. Pictures help visitors focus. I kept going back to the picture in the blue tutu. Like the pine casket she was later buried in, Alyssa's life was simple then. Clear. Straightforward. Happy.

I stood in the hallway waiting for a long time. It was not my place to rush them. Leaving Alyssa would feel like a betrayal, as if you stopped holding on to the last visible piece of her. But at some point you have to say goodbye. In the casket room, Diane's voice rose and fell in anguish. I spent the time asking the funeral director a few questions. "Why did they have this open viewing time?" This is not traditionally a ritual in Jewish burial. After the *tahara* process, the casket is usually covered and sealed.

The director, with a gentleness that had years of experience behind it, paused: "Families who lose someone special in a disfiguring accident or in a state of physical dismemberment, want and need to say goodbye to a person who looks most like the person they remember, especially when the death is sudden." He was pulling out the memory picture card, but I had one myself, so who was I to argue? There might be some relief for Diane and Roy. They knew that after they left the body, someone would carefully take care of Alyssa, clean her and prepare her properly for burial.

There was some other activity going on down the corridor, a chapel service. Funeral home employees and drivers with black satin yarmulkes placed awkwardly on their heads were ready with an easy sympathy to move the proceedings of another sad farewell along. One of them stood just outside the building, leaning against the white brick exterior, having his last smoke before the guests walked outside.

While I had the funeral director's attention, I wanted to understand the appeal of the vault burial. He explained that when water tables are high, people often opt for burial in vaults to prevent the early decomposition of the body. Even those who get buried in the ground must by law have a concrete slab sealer over the casket to ensure that the body stays where it is placed. Other people opt for embalming and some opt for both.

"So how long does the body last when you're embalmed?"

"It can last for a hundred or two hundred years."

"Why would someone want to do that?" I asked aloud, while thinking, *Are we so afraid of not being that we postpone it? Could it be that we are still in denial even after we die?*

"I don't know," he replied. I heard a lot of "I don't knows" in those few days.

Mary Roach in *Stiff*, her famous book on cadavers, observes that undertakers used to tell everyone that sealed vaults and embalming fluids were permanent ways to preserve the body. I'm glad that "my" undertaker did not lie to me. Two hundred years is a long time, but it is not forever. Roach helped me understand the lie through a lawsuit she shared in her book. A man whose mother died bought space in a mausoleum; every six months he would bring his lunch to the cemetery and open his mother's casket for a visit. One rainy spring he came for his biannual visit to find that his mother had grown a beard—a mold beard. He sued the mortuary for $25,000 and since then—excuse the pun—mum's the word on forever.[8]

You can't really check on a dead body's decomposition, at least legally, so all you get for your embalming fee is the mental assurance that you have done your best to keep the worms and the water away for a little longer, not to mention putting off the "earth to earth" biblical injunction. I noticed on the Costco website and other online casket stores that a variation of the following warning appears in bold, almost like the warning on cigarette packages, in case you didn't already know that smoking can kill you: THERE IS NO SCIENTIFIC OR OTHER EVIDENCE THAT ANY CASKET WITH A SEALING DEVICE WILL PRESERVE HUMAN REMAINS. Every time you click "Add item" to your online death cart, this warning appears. No store wants to be responsible for your delusions of eternity.

The warning sums up a fantasy and a repeated theme of unhappy endings. The warning is really about the denial of death. A dead body decomposes. It can be vaulted, embalmed, sealed or preserved in any number of chemical fluids, but any method will just delay the inevitable. Happier endings come to those willing to accept the grim reality of what happens to the body. They come to terms with endings, or at least the end of this life as we know it. They're not trying to outlive nature by fooling themselves.

When the funeral director left, I directed my attention down the hall to the chapel. Watching another funeral take place while you are putting details together for the one you are "hosting" has an odd, stagehand-from-Hades feel to it. I watched the theatrics of the mourning process as I waited for Diane and Roy to emerge from the casket room. Short, older couples—hey, this is Florida—walked out with their heads bowed, the women holding tissues, the men searching pockets for car keys. Funeral employees stood in various places direct-ing traffic and offering hushed words of consolation.

"Sorry for your loss. The parking lot is straight ahead."

"May his memory be for a blessing. The parking lot is straight ahead."

"The parking lot is directly ahead of you. So sorry for your loss."

There was a script here, and the actors had clearly done this show a thousand times before.

One scholar has called the modern funeral a kind of performance art that is closer to Hollywood than it is to any religious practice. We buy into the theater of it and the conventions that come with theat-rics, however hollow or distinguished they might be. Death can be done any way a client's family chooses, but not really—it's any way that the family is directed to choose by morticians who present their wares to vulnerable customers. Tom Jokinen, who wrote *Curtains*, the memoir/exposé of working as an undertaker-in-training, interviewed an owner of three funeral homes in Milwaukee who told him that a funeral is a show. He even tells his staff when he sees a family walk in the door, "It's *Riverdance* time." At his homes they serve food and drinks at visitations: "We are not in the funeral business; we are in the hospitality business."[9]

Mitford discovered the same sales pitch elsewhere when she met a funeral director and mortuary school graduate who described a fu-neral as an odyssey:

> I welcome the family as I would guests to my own home. I offer the rest room, soda, and hospitality. Today, I'd come out with embalming, dressing, visitation. At the end of the arrangements conference, we hold hands, say a prayer, have coffee. I'm a tour guide! . . . We must *all* be tour guides.[10]

This ebullient approach has a great deal to do with the loss of a religious public who would, until only decades ago, have followed whatever practices were conventional within their faith tradition and house of worship. Families today are told that they have choices when it comes to death and that church practices need not hamper their individual style. The problem is that when it comes to death, most people don't have an individual style. The spiritual writer Bruce Feiler observed in his own creation of mourning rituals that the "elaborate, carefully staged mourning rituals" of the past are rarely observed today. "Old customs no longer apply, yet new ones have yet to materialize."[11] What doesn't seem to work is the bumper sticker one hip, young funeral director has on his car: "Let's Put the 'Fun' Back in Funeral."

Max Rivlin-Nadler, the founder of *Full Stop* magazine, describes his visit to the 130th National Funeral Directors' Conference. He saw a new breed of hearses and walked through a hallway of coffins. He saw a makeover using a cosmetics line for the dead being applied to an older woman—who was still alive. "No one seemed to consider this odd or in poor taste. Why would they? To those in the business of death, the distinction between the living and the dead is a simple matter of economics."[12] Rivlin-Nadler learned about a new iPhone app that lets you know the progress of a cremation and went to a "Funeral Directors Under 40: A Night on the Town" event. Someone he met at the event tried to prepare him for the evening and said, lowering his voice, "Funeral directors are notoriously heavy drinkers. There will definitely be some hookups."

While it all sounds strange to the novice, death is an industry like any other. It has its conferences and trade publications. And it also has a new role: to fill in the gaping holes left in the absence of accepted faith traditions. Jokinen believes that the religious practices that have been eclipsed by personal style have often resulted in a hodgepodge ceremony. This kind of theater is weak on substance and high on cliché:

> Take God out of the picture. What's left? The sucking void is still there. How do we fill it? With sacred customs, or by picking and choosing the best from the lot and adapting them for the occasion: a bit of Zen, a touch of Zoroastrianism, yes to candles, no to Psalm 23, a clown, a puppy, show tunes, trained doves released at the gravesite to symbolize the flight of the soul, or whatever else reflects the unique life lost. We're no longer a marginally organized tribe of believers, but a marginally organized tribe of individuals, where each life story is as important as the next.[13]

To that end, human beings become defined less by their faith and convictions and more by their hobbies. So you can get golf-themed plates for a casket and urns shaped like fish for the ashes of the avid fisherman. You can have a gardening theme or a teddy bear for the infant death. The summation of a human life is reduced to whatever keeps us busy for a few hours on a weekend. There is no larger purpose or grander scale to the end of a life. It boils down to what you do in your leisure time.

This trend is not at all surprising if you compare it to sociological trends in virtually every other area of American life. In *Habits of the Heart*, a bestseller about individualism and commitment in the United States, the authors argue that Americans have come to make sharp distinctions between private and public life, to the detriment of the latter. Fierce individualism has weakened the bonds of community responsibility and the notion of the collective, which results in, among other things, the Disney-themed funeral.

> Viewing one's primary task as "finding oneself" in autonomous self-reliance, separating oneself not only from one's parents but also from

those larger communities and traditions that constitute one's past, leads to the notion that it is in oneself, perhaps in relation to a few intimate others, that fulfillment is to be found. Individualism of this sort often implies a negative view of public life. . . . But on the basis of what we have seen in our observation of middle-class American life, it would seem that this quest for purely private fulfillment is illusory: it often ends in emptiness instead.[14]

Americans, the authors believe, are hurting from self-imposed loneliness and a bankruptcy of meaning that is often conferred by feeling part of a community and something larger than self. When we become our hobbies we promote the self and let go of the transcendence that so often accompanies long-standing, communal participation in rituals. We might supplant the need for religion by being a fan of a sports team or by joining a fraternity or a civic association, but it's not only about being part of any group; it's about being part of a group that holds inherent meaning, that is concerned with goodness, responsibility and moral virtue.

Roy, Diane and I left the funeral home to ponder what else we had to do to prepare for the funeral the next day. It's an odd to-do list, to be sure, and not the kind of thing you want to write down and then check off when the tasks are completed:

- plot—check
- casket—check
- death certificate—check
- schedule funeral—check
- call Social Security office to register a death—check
- order deli platters for the *shiva*—check

Much as a checklist seemed inappropriate, I wanted to make sure we had done everything and that the funeral wouldn't have any obvious missing parts, because I was a novice at this, and there was not a second chance to get it right.

Unless you've been through it before, it's hard to imagine how anyone goes from the heart-wrenching chaos of losing someone you love to organizing a funeral, signing documents and buying a plot. Every minute of every hour people die, yet unless it's the death of someone you love, the rituals and practices that follow death seem like the machinations of a secret society that you were never invited to join.

The small, emotional cushions of rituals aid in the transition from the news of death, especially sudden death, to the burial. At first, it seems like a bad dream that someone else dropped you into without an instruction manual. It can be a very lonely and alienating time, when raw emotion has a head-on collision with resentment and theological anger. It becomes difficult to know what's normal and what has to get done.

The funeral director mentioned that, at some point, we needed to inform any companies that extracted payment in the form of bills from Alyssa that she had died. We also might want to call a local paper to put in an obituary. Wanting to spare my relatives the difficulty of canceling out Alyssa's bureaucratic relationship with the government and utilities, I called the phone and cable companies myself. I expected a little sympathy on the other end. Even a two-word "so sorry" would have worked at this point in my fragility. But the news of Alyssa's death, which felt so enormous in my mental space, was insignificant to those on the other end of the phone. It happens every day, I reminded myself. It happens several times a day, calls like these. To them, she wasn't a person, just a number, another bill, another notification. Another fact.

Hanging up the phone, I felt that Alyssa was rapidly disappearing from the world. And she was. The words of the neuroscientist David Eagleman overwhelmed me: "There are three deaths. The first is when the body ceases to function. The second is when the body is consigned to the grave. The third is that moment, sometime in the future, when your name is spoken for the last time."[15]

Alyssa was certainly not disappearing from the hearts and minds of her family, but her name was quickly erased from the lists of institutions that frame our prosaic daily life. This was a new kind of end to me, and it felt like sandpaper chafing on memory. It only strengthened my resolve to capture Alyssa in the eulogy at the service the next day. I wanted words to bring her back to life if we couldn't have her with us. I wondered how many words it would take to give an accurate picture of Alyssa. Was that the goal? Was it to speak to her or to the others at the funeral? Was it to question the suffering or to say goodbye?

Someone posted the news on Facebook, and a new layer of words cropped up. My remaining cousin's best friend flew in from the East Coast with a pile of printouts from Alyssa's Facebook wall that said how special she was and how she would be missed. Just as she was disappearing in some places, her death was generating communication momentum over the internet. Used to the formal note sent snail mail, I was shocked by this outpouring of cyberlove. The internet has changed the way that grieving families help others learn about a death and respond to it. Danna Black, an owner of the company Shiva Sisters, which plans Jewish funerals in Los Angeles, comments on the use of the internet in modern grieving: "If the griever feels comfortable sending out an e-mail, you can feel comfortable sending one back. Just don't Reply All."[16]

My aunt flipped through the pile, stooped over with tears to comment on how nice it was to hear from Alyssa's childhood friends and co-workers, many of whom Diane had never met. These cybervisits were oddly comforting, and they raised a new set of questions: what happens to all our passwords, our eBay account and our social media networks when we go? An iPod user wrote in to an Apple magazine recently to ask whether or not she could bequeath her iTunes collection (of which she was clearly proud) to someone after she's gone. She said she doesn't expect to die anytime soon but thought it a reasonable question. The answer is no: your highly individualized embrace of technology is so highly individualized that you're taking it with you when you go. Perhaps this is why a friend of mine told me that she wants her cellphone to be thrown into the casket when they lower her down. Really? I was actually looking forward to the peace and quiet.

No one wanted to speak at the funeral—or, more correctly, no one else thought they *could* speak at the funeral. No matter how uncomfortable you feel, speak at the funeral of a loved one if given the opportunity, or create the opportunity with a memorial service. No one at a funeral is expecting family members to be eloquent or dry-eyed. Go ahead and cry. The release of tears and the choking actually help listeners appreciate what this person meant to you, and this helps others release their emotions as well. Your speaking from the heart grants permission for everyone to be in that vulnerable place with you. Jewish tradition has an expression: "Words that leave the heart enter the heart." They leave the heart of one and enter the heart of another. There are few regrets worse than "I wish I would have said my final goodbyes and told everyone what my mother really meant to me. There's nothing I can do now." You never get that opportunity again.

I interviewed my remaining cousin and then my aunt and uncle to understand what they regarded as quintessentially Alyssa and what they thought had to be said as we sent her off. Suddenly capturing and summarizing a whole life in a few minutes seemed both urgent and impossible. And then I thought of the noonday sun in Florida and wondered if, on our checklist, we had told the cemetery staff to put up a tent. If not, I'd cut short my remarks. Speaking longer would not necessarily honor her life more.

Diane and Roy didn't want an obituary for Alyssa. They mourned her privately. They weren't looking for attention. They wanted it all to be over. A friend suggested that the family take tranquilizers for the funeral. They wanted to numb the pain. It is well known that people who medicate themselves have a harder time recovering. If you don't confront the pain fully it is harder to get on the other side of it, even if you never really get on the other side of it. My aunt and uncle decided against it. Bob Deits in *Life After Loss* suggests that if you take a tranquilizer at a funeral it prevents you from being as aware as possible of what is happening around you and what your own emotional state is.[17] That day, there was a high level of awareness.

It started to rain just as the funeral was beginning. The ushers held open wide golf umbrellas. For the family, the rain didn't matter. God was crying with us, on us. We pushed the simple pine casket through the gray drizzle, slowly moving it on a roller bed over the wet earth. The ushers lowered the casket to the wails of onlookers. Following Jewish custom, everyone under the tent was asked to shovel a clod of earth into the opening. The family tossed in dirt from Jerusalem's Mount of Olives. We read Psalm 23 together. "Yea, though I walk through the valley of the shadow of death, I will fear no evil, for Thou art with me." I spoke about Alyssa, how easy it was for her to love. Her big heart. Her willingness to forgive. We said the *El Maleh Rachamim* prayer, "God Who is Full of Compassion": "Lord of mercy, bring her under the cover of Thy wings, and let her soul be bound up in the bond of eternal life." I asked for a moment of silence so that each person could ask for Alyssa's forgiveness. We recited another psalm. My then ninety-six-year-old grandmother came late, pushing her walker in the rain. She interrupted the service with a loud cry: "Put me in instead. Take me."

I tried to ignore the outcry and keep going, but my grandmother was right on some level. It makes logical sense in the world of reason for old people to die and young people to live. But I couldn't let the weight of her words derail the ceremony. I quoted from the book of Job. I asked anyone who wanted to share a last word with Alyssa to come up and place a flower in the grave and share a piece of their brokenness with her. There was silence, utter silence, and no movement whatsoever. Slowly, one person rose, took a flower and let out a cry. More people came up. We used up all the flowers.

I prayed with the group of mourners that we allow Alyssa, in her death, to show us how to love. And then I took a deep breath: "Alyssa, teach us to say 'I love you' more often because it came so easy to you. It's not always so easy for us. Teach us how to show deep emotion because it came so easy to you. Teach us not to blame each other for what we didn't give you but to take care of each other because that's what you would have wanted."

We said the *Kaddish*, a Jewish affirmation of life that never mentions death. Leon Wieseltier's words in his book *Kaddish* kept ringing in my ear: magnified and sanctified. Magnified and sanctified. I wished Alyssa farewell and finished my remarks: "Goodbye, fallen angel." It was not clear what to do next, how to end the service. We were stuck in space and time, immobilized by the gravity and awkwardness of it all. I could not ask anyone to leave.

Just then the director whispered in my ear that another service was about to begin. The family was frozen in the front row, under the movable tent. No one wanted Alyssa to be alone. Each member of the family wanted to be the last to go home. My cousin asked if he could put a letter in before they finished the burial, as the bulldozer moved in with its monster claws. The note fluttered down on top of the dirt from the Mount of Olives.

Cars turned on their lights and windshield wipers as the rain cleared. I moved my aunt and uncle into the car, one slow footfall after another. Diane wept in the backseat. "I don't want everyone to come over now. I don't want to see anyone." And I knew exactly what she meant. "Diane, they'll all be there when you get home, even if you don't want them. Some of them may already be there. It's what friends do. They'll be there for you. They also need to grieve."

We arrived at the house and took out the memorial candle that would burn for seven days. I took the cardboard mourners' chairs — reinforced, of course, since mourners come in all shapes and sizes — which are lower than regular chairs, out of the trunk where the director had put them during the service. The dining-room table was covered with platters of cold cuts. People were already eating when my aunt and uncle sat down. I prepared the ritual bread and boiled eggs that symbolize life and put the plate before Diane and Roy. They couldn't eat.

The next days were filled with people. My aunt and uncle passed in and out of the reverie of loss. With each new visitor there was a little punch of new anguish as the story got repeated and the unanswered questions mounted like an emotional landfill. The *shiva* ended. The candle burned out. The guests left. The hurt stayed.

Alyssa's death raised so many questions for me about death. I saw the way that religion helps the dying and the survivors with rituals that cushion liminal time, that in-between time when you experience the first shock of death but have not made headway through death's many stages. What did people do who did not have these rituals? Could they still have a happy ending? I'm not so sure. I thought about the role of friends and community as a safety net for those who survive the worst deaths. Could someone who dies alone have a happy ending? Yes. Alyssa's seemed to be a meaningful end. I watched how our memories sift through the bad like an emotional sieve that leaves us mostly with the residual good. Could we harbor resentment toward the dying and still believe that the death represents a happy ending? I think so. I thought a lot about money and death and how the "property invest-ments" we make for burials, far in advance of when we'll need them, help keep our families whole even when we feel desperate. Can you have a happy ending when you don't make any burial plans? Possibly, but it makes it much harder. Can you have a happy ending without someone to usher you through death? Possibly, but I realized how important it is to have a guide or an escort through the experience, since the practical and theological keep collapsing on each other when it comes to death. I also understood the vacuum that a death like Alyssa's left, a crater-size bowl of sadness that seemed like it would never go away. Would the pain ever depart with the departed? I had questions that needed answers. I had homework to do.

I also realized something new about love during those long days. For survivors, love *is* the afterlife. It's the wounds that suddenly dissipate be-cause you'd trade all of them in for a few more minutes with someone you love. It's the way that the deceased stamp themselves all over the living, in little gestures, in expressions they would have said, in the ex-pectation that when you turn the corner in a familiar space, you will see them again. It's what Rilke called a shooting star in his poem "Death":

> *O shooting star*
> *That fell into my eyes and through my body—*
> *Not to forget you. To endure.*[18]

Where I had so many questions, Diane had one. Where is Alyssa? Diane's curiosity about the afterlife was not intellectually motivated.

She wanted to know if Alyssa was still out there. The thought that her existence—on any level—was truly over was too unbearable.

Every day for the next month I spoke to Diane. Every day, she repeated her question: "Where is her soul now?"

"I don't know," I replied. "I think it's with you."

# Chapter Two

# Pondering the Afterlife

I could not easily let go of Diane's question: what happens to the soul after death? I gave her an answer of sorts, but what if it was a wrong answer in a universe where there are no wrong answers because no one really knows? If my search for a better death had any meaning, I would have to research the afterlife question right away. What happens to us after we die? We ask this question as if it had a simple scientific answer, like the question "Why do people get goosebumps?" or "What is a cloud made of?"

People who believe that a better life awaits us after this one would appear to have secured a happier ending, even before they come close to the end. There is little to be afraid of if you're armed with the promise of a wonderful future. Death is only a portal to greater joy.

When we think of reincarnation, we usually imagine it as an opportunity to have another life with which to learn to play the saxophone or live in Antarctica or keep pet chinchillas. In other words, reincarnation is essentially one more opportunity to do something we always wanted to do but couldn't accomplish in just one lifetime. In the immortal words of Harry Potter's headmaster, Albus Dumbledore: "To the well-organized mind, death is but the next great adventure."

Alternatively, the afterlife is a long retirement vacation where we get a rest from all the havoc of life and work's exertions. With the same daily schedule and appearance of a high-end Club Med vacation, we imagine the afterlife as an exotic tropical location where nothing costs real money and flights are always on time. We find a mental spot on the beach with soft white sand and a few palm trees. We have enough reading material to get us through an eternity; in the afterlife, all the books we read have been positively reviewed. We enjoy girlie drinks with fun names. We tan but need no sunscreen; there is no sunburn in the netherworld. My personal afterlife looks a lot like the Ritz-Carlton in Puerto Rico, complete with royal blue umbrellas and thick, fluffy towels. I can accept that some people need hammocks in their next-life postcard, but being tangled in what looks like a horizontal macramé plant-holder is not part of my afterlife bliss. I'm just not that coordinated. A friend pictures the afterlife as a place of fluffy clouds and Socrates playing chess, and that seems closer to what would work for me if I knew how to play chess.

Mark Twain in *Letters from the Earth* writes that each person imagines himself in a heaven that is basically a variation of his world now: "Heaven is like himself: strange, interesting, astonishing, grotesque. I give you my word, it has not a single feature in it that he *actually values*. It consists—utterly and entirely—of diversions which he cares next to nothing about, here in the earth, yet is quite sure he will like them in heaven."[1] Twain highlights our naïve and limited imaginations. The afterlife will just be a more pleasant version of this life: a great view minus the telephone poles.

The Pew Forum on Religion and Public Life found that 74 percent of Americans believe in some form of life after death. This may be highly correlated with strong religious beliefs among Americans generally.[2] The number goes down globally but is still at a high of 51 percent. The Ipsos Social Research Institute conducted a poll of 18,000 people from 23 countries and found that just over half of them believe in an afterlife, with only 23 percent believing that we just cease to exist after we die. Roughly a quarter of us have no idea what will happen after we die. When it comes to the afterlife, skeptics are in the minority.

These results may cohere with the two choices Socrates put before us: "Death is one of two things. Either it is annihilation, and the dead have no consciousness of anything; or, as we are told, it is really a change: a migration of the soul from one place to another." Since we have no idea what happens, and we'd rather opt for the migration of souls than for annihilation, the afterlife looks more promising—especially as we creep closer to the estimated time of departure. The poet Allen Ginsberg is reported to have said often: "I don't have proof that there is reincarnation, but I must give it the benefit of the doubt, because if there is, and I have to go through it, I should be ready; I don't want to miss the opportunity to help myself."[3] None of us wants to miss out on that. But if the statistics are right, 26 percent of us aren't so sure.

In reality, the afterlife is the next great unexplored frontier. The problem is that no one has been there and back. But apparently, some people claim to have gotten a closer look than others. A Gallup Poll conducted in 1982 concluded that one in every twenty Americans has had at least one near-death experience (NDE).[4] By analyzing thousands of near-death experiences, Dr. Jeffrey Long postulated in *Evidence of the Afterlife* that NDEs stimulate thoughts about God, forgiveness, love, hardships and purpose and are "strikingly consistent across cultures, races and creeds."[5] His findings were derived from collecting NDEs across the world on his website www.nderf.org/afterlife. Below are the most salient features of NDEs he identified:

1. Separation of consciousness from the physical body, popularly called an out-of-body experience
2. Heightened or highly alert senses
3. Intense feelings or emotions that are generally positive
4. Vision of a tunnel, often with the experience of traveling through the tunnel
5. Vision of bright light or being wrapped with a bright light
6. Encounter with deceased relatives, friends or mystical beings
7. A sense of alteration of time and/or space
8. Life review of major events or relationships
9. Encounter with otherworldly realms
10. Gain of special knowledge
11. Confrontation with a boundary, particularly one that directs a person back to her body and previous life
12. A return to the body, sometimes willingly or unwillingly[6]

The image of moving toward the light through a tunnel-like passage is a common feature of NDEs, and even people who know little about such experiences have seen this image in movies like the popular 1990s film *Flatliners* or have read about it in books.

NDEs helped reshape attitudes about living for those who experienced them. The overarching finding of Long's work was that having an NDE helped people accept and even welcome death. NDEs also changed their thoughts about living and relationships:

Patients with an NDE did not show any fear of death, they strongly believed in an afterlife, and their insight into what is important in life had changed: love and compassion for oneself, for others and for nature. They understood the cosmic law that everything one does to others will ultimately be returned to oneself: hatred and violence as well as love and compassion.[7]

The payback impulse was heightened for those who have had NDEs because they got a glimpse of what to expect from the afterlife. They came back to this life with a "do-over" mentality. Kenneth Ring, in *Heading Toward Omega: In Search of the Meaning of the Near-Death Experience,* concluded that those who had a near-death experience had greater self-confidence, a stronger sense of spirituality, decreased materialism and a renewed love of life.[8]

Long's list makes death more palatable for the living who have experienced NDEs in part because death is like one big family reunion. Being reunited with ancestors is part of the common parlance of death. We talk about dead relatives smiling down on us at special milestones or those near death dreaming about the moment when they will once again see a beloved spouse or child who died before them, but for those with NDEs, these encounters seem real. This belief provides solace when facing death, and this feature of the NDE—perhaps more than any other—is shared across many spiritual traditions.

Many faiths stress that the afterlife begins with an in-gathering of family members we profoundly miss. When Abraham, the first patriarch of the Hebrew Bible, died, Genesis records his happy ending in just this way: "And Abraham breathed his last, dying at a good, ripe age, old and contented; and *he was gathered to his ancestors*" (Genesis 25:8). Isaac, Abraham's son and heir, died in similar fashion: "He was *gathered to his kin* in ripe old age" (Genesis 35:29). Jacob, Isaac's son, gave his last will and testament and then left his universe of suffering and difficulty: "When Jacob finished his instructions to his sons, he drew his feet into the bed, breathing his last, *he was gathered to his people*" (Genesis 49:33). These deaths communicate that the end is a passage to family reunification, usually in the presence of living family members. Similarly, in ancient teachings of Buddhist tradition, death is a time when you are gathered up with your ancestors, who escort you to the next stage of life. Ancient texts aside, we often hear people speak about the next world in just this way: "Now Uncle Ed can finally join Aunt Bessie. She's been waiting for him." And it sounds as if heaven is not Uncle Ed's destination. Instead he's going to a family picnic, and he's really, really late.

NDEs confirmed, for those who had experienced them, that there is an afterlife and that the next life offers something rich and meaningful to look forward to when this life is over. But the skeptic in me was still struggling. I had never met anyone who had a near-death experience or would, in my social circles, admit to having had one. And then one Sunday morning while trolling the newspapers, I came across Dan Leviton's obituary. Leviton taught a thanatology class in the health department of the University of Maryland for over thirty years and inducted hundreds of students into a deliberative process of facing a reality that most people ignore entirely. He spent his professional life making the world a better place by teaching people how to die. When he joined the university in the 1960s, he was one of only a few professors in the country who taught thanatology, and one of his main objectives was to help students confront the fear of death and, thereby, to overcome it.

His obit contained praise from former students whose lives had been shaped by Leviton's teachings. I decided to reach out to one of them, only later to find out that Carolyn was not only one of his prize students. Her experience in Leviton's courses helped her piece together the meaning of an NDE that actually saved her life and helped her heal the deep scars of a bruised childhood. I finally found someone who had a near-death experience and was willing to talk about it.

Carolyn came to the University of Maryland from Canada as a young adult, leaving a small college in Montreal to study exercise science and aging in the States, specifically cardiac rehabilitation; this degree was not offered anywhere in Canada at the time. She described herself as a young, shy and unsophisticated graduate student who was afraid to raise her hand in class. Carolyn was deeply committed to preventative medicine, but she struggled with the difference in values she experienced in America: "People just don't understand how different a social democracy is from a capitalist society." The university atmosphere was a far cry from what Carolyn was used to at home.

Carolyn grew up with strict Italian parents in a Catholic home whose cultural clock measured time in Catholic holidays. She had never seen drugs before but had seen a lot of drinking; she didn't understand some of the cultural norms in the United States and felt that people were much more lackadaisical about their health. Where some people might view these problems as merely social differences, Carolyn experienced them as personal losses: loss of country, loss of language, loss of faith.

Carolyn met Professor Dan Leviton in her first semester and decided to take part in a course he was offering on intergenerational adult health and development, allowing her the opportunity to work with aging adults. It was a chance to talk about death and loss with people who were much closer to it than she was. "They came for companionship and in return showed the students how to age."[9]

Carolyn found herself writing about her losses in his class, and Leviton encouraged her to explore them. Now in her midfifties,

Carolyn has come to believe that death is just one of many types of grief on a scale of pain that includes rejection, abandonment, unemployment and retirement. She currently has a sixteen-year-old son with regressive autism, and she talks slowly and mournfully about the life that her son will never have. And it becomes yet another loss. She experienced this as anxiety, having lost fourteen pounds in the past year: "I held so much grief in my body. I just couldn't eat."

In those first graduate school years, Leviton needed an assistant for his aging program, and he liked Carolyn. As an agnostic Jew, he praised his young Catholic graduate student for her openness. Leviton was a compassionate skeptic who wanted his students to appreciate the complexity of end-of-life issues. Carolyn remembers an eighty-year-old vet in the program whom one graduate student was prodding to give up smoking. "Dan just told him to leave the guy alone. The withdrawal at his age could hurt him more." At the peak of the program, Dan and his students were a staff of ninety working with about sixty older adults. Carolyn worked with him for twelve years.

Dan always ran the seminar on death; he was very blunt with his students, who would often come to his house to discuss it. This helped Carolyn process, for the first time, many difficult aspects of her childhood: "I had a lot of experience with death. As Catholics, we were carted off to funeral homes all of the time. When I was five, my great-grandmother passed away, and I remember picking up her arm in the coffin to have her wave bye-bye. I saw one of my aunts, who lost her husband, jump into the grave, she was so bereft." Carolyn's childhood was filled with memories of going to people's homes who had lost someone and seeing them inconsolable. "All the community would come out. Italians who only spoke Italian. Italians who only spoke English."

She was ten when President Kennedy was shot, and because he was Catholic the entire parochial school system closed. Fascinated by what she calls "old country grief," she found it hard to understand Jackie Kennedy's stoic approach. Kennedy's wife was not crying the way her mother and grandmother were crying. "And we weren't even American!"

Carolyn then spoke slowly, measuring each word. Something important was on her mind. "You know . . . as a child . . . it did cross my mind to take my own life." I had not expected the conversation to go in this direction. Carolyn's parents were very punitive and believed in corporal punishment. "I was a curious and spirited child. I got hit a lot with wooden spaghetti sticks that broke in half over you. Today we call it child abuse. Back then you called it discipline."

Her voice became even slower, more quiet: "It took its toll on me. I was very, very sad. It occurred to me to just check out of the misery I was in. I felt trapped. I knew there was something else to life that I wasn't getting." We sat in the silence of Carolyn's pain for a moment. She confessed to never having told anyone this.

"What stopped you from taking your life?"

Her answer caught me off guard.

At the age of ten, before any of the current literature we have on NDEs was out, Carolyn had a near-death experience. She had repressed the memory totally until Dan Leviton's class on near-death experiences, but she had not repressed the emotions of the experience, and it was these emotions that saved her.

I was in Atlantic City at the beach with my parents, and there had been a hurricane. We were in the ocean in the aftermath of the hurricane. I could swim, but my parents couldn't. I was holding my dad's hand and jumping in the waves. Suddenly there was a huge surge, and it knocked us all down. I thought I had died. And then I was in the presence of God, this force. There was a tunnel of light or a prism—it was narrow and then it got wider. There is no word to describe the whiteness of this light. It was peaceful. As I got closer and closer, the light was pulling me in and becoming bigger.

Carolyn shared this memory almost matter-of-factly, as if the light she saw then was something familiar and close even now. Carolyn is not alone in her recollections. Light plays an important role in most NDEs, and her experience had many of the classic elements that Long describes, including its emotional aftermath. She saw intense light as she was sinking underwater. Only later did she understand that she was close to death at the time.

> I was actually drowning, but that's not what I felt. I had this feeling that being Carolyn and being a girl left me. I did not have parents. I didn't have gender or age. I was just a being enveloped by love. It was a feeling you can't even describe. After being married and having children and loving children, I still cannot imagine loving anything the way I loved that light and the way I felt loved by it. The first thing I said when I came to was, "Leave me alone. I want to go back." My father remembers me saying this.

Carolyn's father pulled her hair to get her out of the water and then deposited her on the beach. She came to and vomited saltwater and cried her eyes out. Her parents made her lie down on a blanket on the sand to calm her down. No one asked her about the experience. At ten, she did not have the language to articulate or process it. No one recognized it as a trauma. She tucked it deep inside.

"The experience made me believe that there is one God and that we are all loved by some sort of Creator." Carolyn compared her experience to the description St. Teresa of Avila used to describe the soul as a place of many rooms. Depending on your spiritual level, you might be far from God, but you can also become closer and experience God at closer range. This is what Carolyn believes happened to her: "I was invincible because I was so protected. I was in a different world. I was loved beyond imagination. I felt more and more heat as I got closer and closer; I was more enveloped by this love. And I heard music, what sounded like angels singing. It may have been my religious conditioning, but that's what it sounded like to me."

Carolyn felt light and happy, elation. "It was euphoria. 'Be still and know that I am'—if I had to put my adult spin on what happened to me, that's it." When her father jerked her out of the water, he also jerked her out of the experience, and she returned to her ten-year-old body. She is, forty-five years later, still afraid of the ocean. But she is not afraid of death, and her experience then emotionally rescued her from putting an end to her misery.

Carolyn affirmed what the research bears out: those who believe in the afterlife are better prepared for death and less frightened by it. But how many of us truly believe that there is a life after this one? For a minority of us, even people of faith, the universe of science has blunted our capacity to accept that there is a life after this one. Our resident death expert, Kübler-Ross, says that our society has shifted from a religious orientation that offered a belief in the afterlife to an increasingly secular society that denies death by putting a premium on youth. This shift has generated greater anxiety by denying people ultimate hope and purpose, the kind that literally saved Carolyn's life.[10] Kübler-Ross believes our denial and fear of death—in the absence of religious belief in the world to come—have contributed to increasing violence and destructiveness and the urge "to kill in order to avoid the reality of facing of our own death."[11]

Most Jews and Christians I know believe in God or some transcendent force outside themselves and may even go to a house of worship regularly, but when pressed they will say: "I'm not sure there's an afterlife." The burden of skepticism overwhelms many. Even were we to conclude that belief in the afterlife helps people have a happier ending, it doesn't mean that you can foist that belief onto a questioning mind with no concrete proof. Many of us go through life with an unarticulated hope discussed by philosophers as a religious gambit: if there is life after death, and we have been morally upright or religiously believing, then we will be rewarded with heaven; if not, there has been little harm in a life lived with faith.

F. W. H. Myers did not appreciate this kind of speculation. Why make life feel like a wager if you could create the kind of scientific schemata to know with certainty if life exists after this one? Myers (1843–1901) was a spiritualist and head of the Society for Psychical Research, as it was called in the nineteenth century. For decades, he had been a school inspector in Cambridge, England, but had a transformational moment in 1869 when Henry Sidgwick provoked him to consider life after this one during an evening walk. Sidgwick (1838–1900) was an English philosopher and economist. He was no stranger to faith; his father was a reverend by profession. Sidgwick went on to lecture at Cambridge. Together, Myers and Sidgwick co-led the society and were able, because of their intellectual credentials, to persuade others to join them, including such eminent contemporaries as Charles Darwin, Francis Galton and George Eliot.

With radical, fanatic ambition driving him, Myers believed that the great scientific minds of the day should investigate—using their tools of reason—whether there was indeed life after death. In his words, "If all attempts to verify scientifically the intervention of another world should be definitely proved futile, this would be a terrible blow, a mortal blow, to all our hopes of another life, as well as of traditional religion."[12] In other words, if there were truly no afterlife, it may just change everything. It would certainly alter religion dramatically. So

Myers put himself to the task, devoting himself body and soul to figuring out, to the best of his knowledge, if a world exists after this one. He collaborated on the society's first book on the paranormal. Words that now enjoy household use—"telepathy, supernormal, veridical"—were all a gift of Myers. Lest we think that he was just a quack with greater sophistication than your average charlatan, William James, the founder of psychology, suggested that the problems of the subliminal mind should be called "the problem of Myers." And he added, "Whatever the judgment of the future may be on Mr. Myers' speculation, the credit will always remain to him of being the first attempt in any language to consider the phenomena of hallucination, automatism, double personality, and mediumship as connected parts of one whole subject."[13]

Myers created a metaphysical language to begin any and all conversations about life after death. And he legitimized the participation of intellectuals in matters generally regarded as beneath them, including the likes of Sigmund Freud, Carl Jung, William Butler Yeats, Aldous Huxley and others.

The movement petered out when Myers died, but he had opened the door to the scientific study of what is generally considered unknowable. John Gray in his book on this unusual group, *The Immortalization Commission: Science and the Strange Quest to Cheat Death*, describes a telling moment in the history of this society. When Myers died in Rome in 1901, his friend William James sat in a nearby room close to its open door, with a pen in hand and his notebook on his knees, to share cross-correspondence with Myers. The page remained blank.[14]

Myers is now gone, and aside from psychics on summer boardwalks and in Bruce Springsteen songs, there's not much cross-correspondence any more. Maybe afterlife texting?

Today, the people who have most closely mimicked Myers's experiments and interests are those who have had near-death experiences and come back to this world to talk about them. Myers and his cohorts may have given us a lexicon of terms but never proved with scientific accuracy what happens after we die. Yet language does shape experience. Just ask Carolyn. She sat in Dan Leviton's class fifteen years after her near drowning, listened to him speak about NDEs and heard herself exclaim: "Oh my God. That happened to me." The fact that it happened before all the literature came out validated it for her. And Leviton was genuinely interested in what happened to Carolyn. "He called it my woo-woo experience, teasing me. He was really skeptical. He had no patience whatsoever for organized religions because he felt they'd done so much damage. At the same time he actually introduced me to Elisabeth Kübler-Ross and also Robert Kastenbaum, who wrote *the* textbook on the psychology of death." Carolyn went on to complete her doctorate and, like Leviton, has made a career of helping adults confront their health challenges as they age. Like her mentor, Carolyn tried to provide others with a language to speak about the mystery of afterlife experiences that people used to keep to themselves. She frequently taught preretirement seminars on nutrition and health and laughed when she told me of a seminar she ran at the Pentagon. A group of overachieving men, including a one-star general, tolerated her presentation, waiting for her to finish because the speaker after her specialized in retirement financing. They perked up suddenly when she started talking about NDEs. Slowly stories started to surface. There was the Vietnam vet who thought he'd had one, and another man who said he left his body during open-heart surgery and watched the doctors and nurses operate from above. The experience was so vivid that he could say afterward what the ring looked like that a nurse was wearing under her glove. The military men had never shared these stories before. Their near confrontation with death bonded them. Carolyn understood that she needed to create a safe space for people to explore experiences beyond their immediate understanding.

Carolyn also firmly believes the lesson Dan Leviton taught her: you can control the way you die. "I don't know all the factors, but if I put things in place, I will have greater control of my death and make sure that whoever is with me when I take my last breath will respect the essence of who I was." And, for a woman who has been profoundly altered by a mystical experience she cannot fully explain, Carolyn intends to make the same generous offer that her mentor, Dan Leviton, made. When she dies, she wants her body to go to science.

I was less skeptical of NDEs after speaking with Carolyn about hers. I also began to understand the contribution near-death experiences have for the living, the way they fortify people's drive for meaning in this world. The love Carolyn encountered helped her find a greater purpose in life and overcome the darkness immediately in front of her. Her near-death experience transformed her and saved her. But most of us will—thankfully—never come that close to death and return to have this value-added experience. Reading about the NDEs of others made me a little jealous, I have to confess, but it did not make me a believer. And I imagine that most people who have shared the characteristics of a near-death experience did not believe in an afterlife until they had one. It's a little risky to invite people to crash a car and hope they live through it on the slim chance that they will enter a world of light, God and the spiritual equivalent of a family get-together.

In my search for an answer for the skeptic, I found comfort in the guise of neuroscience. The neuroscientist David Eagleman, mentioned earlier, studies time, perception and synesthesia in his lab at Baylor University; in his spare hours, he writes fiction. According to a profile in *The New Yorker,* Eagleman fell off a roof at age eight and felt, after he hit the ground, that he kept falling. Since then, he has collected hundreds of stories of people in life-threatening situations, where time seems to stand still or slow down significantly. He is fascinated by time. For months he wore a broken watch to work. One day—while wearing his watch—he asked someone in his lab what time it was, only to find out that his colleagues also did not wear functioning watches. It was a lab full of people studying time, all of whom were wearing broken watches. "Scientists are often drawn to things that bedevil them," he said. "I know one lab that studies nicotine receptors, and all the scientists are smokers, and another lab that studies impulse control, and they're all overweight."[15]

Eagleman's interest in time may have prompted him to write *Sum: Forty Tales from the Afterlives,* reimagining in short essays what the afterlife might be. In one essay, Eagleman envisions the afterlife as a place where you visit all of the other possible lives you could have led had you made different decisions. You are judged not against other people but against the self you might have been. At first, seeing alternate "yous" makes you feel pride, like the pride you feel in a family member who is successful. You feel attached even remotely to that person's sense of accomplishment. This feeling, however, does not last:

> These yous are not really you, they are better than you. They made smarter choices, worked harder, invested the extra effort into pushing on closed doors. . . . Such success cannot be explained away by a better genetic hand; instead, they played your cards better. In their parallel lives, they made better decisions, avoided moral lapses, did not give up on love so easily. They worked harder than you did to correct

their mistakes and apologized more often. . . . You discover you've never felt more competitive with anyone in your life.[16]

Eagleman's imagined kind of death is the ultimate punishment, because falling short of your potential is spelled out in the clearest way as you encounter all those yous you could have been.

Eagleman's story made me think of the famous Hasidic tale of Rabbi Meshulam Zusha of Hanipol (1718–1800), otherwise known as Reb Zusha. Rabbi Zusha used to say, "When I die and come before the heavenly court, if they ask me, 'Zusha, why were you not Abraham?' I'll say that I didn't have Abraham's intellectual abilities. If they say, 'Why were you not Moses?' I'll say I didn't have Moses' leadership abilities. For every such question, I'll have an answer. But if they say, 'Zusha, why were you not Zusha?' for that, I'll have no answer."

Eagleman's story and Zusha's wisdom raise the critical question of why we need the afterlife. Often we want to believe in an afterlife because we need it. We need to believe there is more to life than what we experience. Like some thrilling roller-coaster ride that only lasts for a few minutes, we can't believe it's over. We believe in second chances and nine lives, that we can be different in some alternate version of the universe. We can have one big predestined do-over and get it right. But perhaps the afterlife can also function like an easy pass in this life. When you get another chance in some far-off future time, you may not think of the consequences of every decision you make now. Eagleman points to consequences in the far-off future that help us redeem the present in a way that only death can. What picture of an invisible future would *you* need to change the present?

Trying to understand if belief in an afterlife helps people overcome their fear of dying, I realized I had to leave my faith comfort zone and explore options outside of the purely secular and academic realms. No religion does afterlife more prominently than Buddhism. Forget Eagleman's consequences. In the Buddhist tradition, if you don't act on goodness and compassion now, you're coming back as an insect. It doesn't get more humiliating than that. Buddhism teaches that there are consequences to each decision you make *here* for the life you will later experience somewhere else. If life has a sequel, as most of us believe it does, then isn't it reasonable to assume there was also a prequel?

Buddhists believe that rebirth creates a different way to approach death, one that radically alters the way we behave in life. Although ancient Buddhist tradition believed that death was a gathering to one's ancestors, the Upanishads replaced that with the tradition of samsara, an endless cycle or circling of death and rebirth. Those unfamiliar with Eastern ideas of death have great difficulty digesting the meaning of reincarnation or its significance. Malcolm David Eckel, a professor of Buddhism at Boston University, remembers approaching a Buddhist monk in India and asking him to divulge if he truly believed in reincarnation. The monk was astonished and asked him if there were really people who *didn't* believe in rebirth.[17]

Gehlek Rimpoche explains how fundamental the idea of rebirth is in his faith: "Reincarnation is something we Tibetans tend to take for granted. We are brought up with the idea that the kind of life we have now is a result of how we have behaved in the past, and that the kind of life we will live in the future depends on how we conduct ourselves now."[18] He believes that rebirth creates greater confidence for the moment when people face death because, if they have made their lives meaningful, they have nothing to fear.[19]

In the Buddhist tradition, the moment of death is exceptionally holy since it marks not only the end of one life but also the beginning of a new life cycle. Most deaths are dramatized with tears and pain, screaming and loss. But in the Buddhist tradition, these behaviors demonstrate attachments that make separation very difficult for the dying. Buddhism focuses less on the anguish of the survivors and more on the leave-taking of the dead and the sanctifying of last breaths. The Dalai Lama emphasizes the importance of the moment of death because it can actually influence the future of the one who is dying: "Although how or where we will be reborn is generally dependent on karmic forces, our state of mind at the time of death can influence the quality of our next rebirth."[20]

I wanted to know how Buddhists achieve this, so I took my search to the top. The Dalai Lama was coming to town, and I decided to seek my own enlightenment at the Verizon Center, where he was praying and teaching for about a week. I was not sure what to wear to my first *Kalachakra,* which in Sanskrit means "time-cycle" and refers to an initiation into the Buddhist tradition. I had nothing in the pumpkin/saffron family so I opted for a vintage red shirt and blazer, only to find that flowing skirts and sandals were more the norm, and that was mostly among the men.

The Verizon Center was hot and stuffed with people. His Holiness was sitting lotus style on an elaborate filigreed throne several feet from the floor surrounded by monks in saffron robes who sat on the floor, flanked on both of his sides. The Dalai Lama was also in a saffron robe with red piping and a matching red visor. Above the stage, large, intricate banners lined the ceiling. There was a wooden ladder leading up to the throne, and from a distance the most powerful figure of contemporary Buddhism looked small. His face was projected on large screens throughout the hall; his smile seemed to inhabit the whole room. On one side of the stage rested a mandala, an intricate sand painting, usually in the shape of a circle inside a square, on a large platform. Over the days that the Dalai Lama was in Washington, he filled in the pattern of the mandala only to have it destroyed by the end of his visit, enacting the impermanence of this life. I hoped that through his teachings I would understand how the impermanence of this world would help me understand the afterlife.

The Dalai Lama, the fourteenth in his line of Gelug Buddhists, is said to be a reincarnation of a previous *lama* or *tulku*. *Lama* is just the Tibetan version of the word "guru" or "great teacher," and the word *dalai* means "ocean," implying the vastness of the Dalai Lama's wisdom. A *tulku* is a very special guru who, by virtue of his spiritual achievements, is allowed to choose the form of his rebirth. This permission is not granted to any other rank of Buddhist. A *tulku* can come back in another gender and as any other type of sentient being. His choice to continue the line of previous *tulkus* is a statement of his responsibility to enlighten his followers.

So here's the dilemma: once the Dalai Lama passes on—and he has already retired from his political position as the head of the Tibetan government in exile—how do his followers identify the one who has been reincarnated to take his place? We can look back at the search for the current Dalai Lama for a clue. The search is called a *yangsi* and is conducted both by officials from the Tibetan government and high-ranking *lamas* of the Gelug School. Usually the next Dalai Lama is from Tibet—but not always. The current Dalai Lama has hinted that his successor may be from outside of Tibet. The search can take several years, leaving Tibetans somewhat leaderless as the transition takes place. It took four years to find the current Dalai Lama, the length of an American presidential term.

The search committee, for lack of a better expression, waits for signs at a special lake where they meditate and have visions. They also watch the direction of the smoke during the cremation of the previous Dalai Lama. This is how they identified Tenzin Gyatso, the birth name of the current Dalai Lama, when he was only a child. The regent or interim leader had a graphic vision of the monastery that housed Tenzin, and then the committee sought out the building that matched that vision. Once they found the boy, the group did a series of tests to confirm his identity. In one, they placed a number of seemingly random objects before him, and because Tenzin chose the objects belonging to the previous Dalai Lama, they knew he was the one. (Interestingly, if there is more than one possible candidate, then the committee places names in an urn and decides through a vote.) Tenzin was deemed the next Dalai Lama and brought with his family to a monastery in Lhasa, where he began years of study and training.

Learning about the process is startling if you imagine trying to identify a future political leader this way. The process underscores just how foundational reincarnation is to the Buddhist tradition, even though to a non-Buddhist it seems quite arbitrary and risky. It's one thing to believe in a loose understanding of *karma* as a long-term payback for things you messed up or did right in this world. It's another to make political appointments of the highest order based on something as ethereal as a vision at a lake and a game with a four-year-old. I brought my question about the risks of reincarnation and leadership to Matteo, a Buddhist, writer and a social activist.

I met Matteo in a teahouse on a sweltering summer day to talk about death. There seemed to be no air-conditioning; perhaps they were trying to simulate the atmosphere of purgatory to inspire atonement. Although Matteo had already written a book on Buddhism, he described himself simply as a practitioner and was excited to share his beliefs with me. He said that death is central to all Buddhist thought, and he explained his morning meditation practice to illustrate the point. That morning, he said, he'd had a little watermelon juice, gone up to the shrine in his home and meditated with the following prayer, which begins with a reflection on Dharma, the state of law or nature:

*First, contemplate the preciousness of being free and well favored.*
*This is difficult to gain, easy to lose;*
*now I must do something meaningful.*
*Second, the whole world and its inhabitants are impermanent;*
*in particular, the life of beings is like a bubble.*
*Death comes without warning; this body will be a corpse.*
*At that time, the Dharma will be my only help;*
*I must practice it with exertion.*
*Third, when death comes, I will be helpless.*
*Because actions bear their inevitable effect,*
*I must abandon evil deeds*
*and always devote myself to virtuous actions.*
*Thinking this every day, I will examine myself.*
*Fourth, attachment to home, friends, wealth,*
*and the comforts of samsara*
*are the constant torments of the three sufferings,*
*Just like a feast before the executioner leads you to your death.*
*I must cut desire and attachment*
*and attain enlightenment through exertion.*
*Recognizing this, may my mind turn toward spiritual practice!*

Matteo, in his prayer, tries to focus on letting go of attachments and contemplating goodness so that he will not fear death, which is the inevitable direction—but not end—of all human life.

Matteo had recently turned forty but looked younger. He lived in Nepal and has been to Tibet more than twenty times. He runs a nonprofit called Nekorpa—meaning "pilgrim" in Sanskrit—that restores and preserves pilgrimage sites damaged by the large volume of traffic from worshipers and tourists to Buddhist holy sites in Nepal, Tibet, Sri Lanka, Mongolia and India. Bemoaning the trash left by visitors, Matteo has tried to help people preserve their spiritual heritage by creating a cleaner, more pleasant experience. Nekorpa provides guidebooks to a number of such sites, and he showed me a postcard of Adam's Peak, a mountain in Sri Lanka that he has climbed many times as an example of a place that his organization is trying to protect. Matteo has also worked for the special envoy to the Dalai Lama and has met His Holiness many times as a result of the work he has done bringing political documents out of Tibet, mostly testimonials to Tibetan suffering at the hands of the Chinese. True to form, he minimizes the significance of his work, but Richard Gere, who wrote the introduction to Matteo's book, *In the Shadow of the Buddha*, calls him "a reliable, skillful, and joyously energized individual" who works on behalf of human rights and religious free-dom.[21]

I asked Matteo if rebirth is considered a gift or a burden in Bud-dhism. He told me that reincarnation is often viewed as a burden, a ceaseless rolling over of responsibility and accountability for one's actions into the life we will next lead. While we tend to use the word "karma" to mean a vibe or a mood in common parlance, in the spiri-tual tradition, karma merely means an act that has consequences. In this way, karma is an extension of justice; acts have consequences that may get played out in another life if they do not get paid out in this one. Gehlek Rimpoche describes the process:

> Enlightened masters . . . stress that negative emotions—anger, at-tachment, hatred and jealousy—are the original cause that keeps us trapped in the cycle of life and death. From negative emotions come negative actions, from negative action comes karma, and from nega-tive karma come karmic consequences.[22]

A popular Buddhist sage regards samsara as a caterpillar moving on a blade of grass. In order to advance, the caterpillar must turn in on itself and then step slowly along, incrementally making its way from one blade of grass to another.

As a spiritual practitioner, Matteo believes that being a Buddhist is always training in the practice of dying, and he shared a popular Buddhist story with me to illustrate *karma* and causality. Siddhartha, the birth name of Gautama Buddha, the founder of Buddhism, came upon a bodhi tree near the hamlet of Gaya. There he vowed not to move from his meditation seat under the tree until he had seen the Truth of reality and understood the source of suffering. That evening, deep in meditation, he saw that all suffering is caused by ignorance of the fact that our existence is in a constant state of flux and that all of our emotions ultimately result in suffering. Siddhartha logically understood that if the cause of suffering were removed, then the effect would not arise—that the cycle of suffering would be broken. The Buddha did not receive anything when he became awakened; quite the contrary, he got rid of what was keeping him from enlightenment. What's more, he said this was possible for all of us.

When death is a source of fear, joy gets replaced with suffering. When the Buddha was asked what nirvana is, he replied that it is the absence of suffering: profound peace. "Dukha" is the Sanskrit word for the feeling of unsatisfactoriness or pervasive discontent, the sensations and actions that separate us from nirvana. Matteo explained that Buddhists study the nature of *dukha* and how to remove it by practicing meditation, ethics, morality and wisdom. Practicing compassion and believing that all things and beings are interconnected removes it. Therefore, when we cause harm to ourselves, we are also causing harm to others. "We must remove that suffering," Matteo said. A belief in life after death could minimize that pain.

In his studies of ancient Buddhist texts, the Vedas and the Upanishads, and more contemporary works, Matteo came to believe that not only is Buddhism distinct from other Eastern religions, but it also seems revolutionary. In death, an autonomous soul finds a new home distinct from the body. In Buddhism there is the corporeal self, the body, and the mind or consciousness, the soul. There is only one thing we know for sure in life, and that is that we're going to die. Everything else you cannot know.

The actual moment of death can be extremely traumatic for the dying and their loved ones, or it can be intensely peaceful. Buddhists believe that if one gains stability and mastery in meditation, a person can actually control what happens to his or her mind at the moment of death. In the Buddhist tradition, there is a transitional stage between the death of the body and the rebirth of the mind called *bardo*, or limbo. It takes three days for consciousness to leave the body. When the mind and body separate there is a moment when true practitioners can stay in the state of pure mind or consciousness. If you are able to do that, then rebirth will not take place because you have entered nirvana, a state beyond suffering.

Matteo told me that his own teacher taught him to have "a genuine heart of sadness" because joy is temporal. He finds himself, like all of us, creating attachments and aversions all of the time. "I make my own sadness," he explains. He can't help himself, he says. But he tries to push his baser thoughts away in the ever-elusive journey toward enlightenment. "No matter what you do you are in charge of your own life." This means that you are also in charge of your own death. You can control your fear. You can end your own suffering or promote it.

Leaving Matteo, I felt liberated, lighter, almost like a burden had been lifted from me. That may have been the result of stepping into an air-conditioned car. But it was also because my talk with him had clarified a lot of the readings I had done in Buddhism for many months, trying to understand something that felt so far from my consciousness. I had a naïve picture of the Buddhist afterlife as a hamster wheel guided by some inexplicable divine force. And if you don't watch yourself carefully you may come back as the actual hamster. What Matteo helped me appreciate was how much we make our own happiness or sadness and how those decisions can have immense long-term consequences, long past our time of death. We stop breathing, but the pulsing of the worlds we created lives beyond us and impacts others.

I brought Matteo's conversation back home, trying to integrate all that I had been learning and thinking about the afterlife. Matteo's observations made one sentence in Maimonides' *Guide to the Perplexed* jump off the page. In this life we are body and soul; the purpose of faith is *tikkun ha-nefesh ve-tikkun ha-guf*, to enhance the body and enhance the soul. We expect Maimonides, as a Jewish physician and philosopher, to believe that a meaningful existence stretches us both physically and metaphysically. But when we die, Maimonides writes elsewhere, the soul is released from the body. If we spend this life working on the physical or material aspects alone—we drive fast cars, look for fast women and eat fast food—then the soul is not nurtured and cannot live beyond us. It dies when we die. But if we do work on the soul in this life, in discovering and promoting the uniqueness that is our purpose, then that soul shines and radiates, and it never dies. And a skeptic may be able to live with that version of the afterlife and the challenge it leaves the living. It would seem to lead to a happier ending.

The Hasidic storyteller and sage Rabbi Nahman once said, "The day you were born was the day God decided that the world could not exist without you." If this is true then actualizing our purpose in this life is the legacy we leave when we die. That legacy lives on in the memories people have of us, in the small things they do that we once did, in the challenges that we gift to them, in the voice that we leave behind that whispers in the ears of our descendants.

And what if you just don't believe that there is anything beyond this life?

You can still believe that there is this life. And this life is not a belief. It is a fact. And in this life, the you that you are may never see the you that you could have been. So why wait for an afterlife? You have tomorrow.

*Chapter Three*

# Sanctifying the Body in Death

M ost of us have never seen a dead body. Why would we? Sherwin Nuland in *How We Die* remarks that the poets and wise men who write about death have rarely seen it, and the doctors and nurses who are everyday witnesses to death rarely write about it.[1] I did not want to see Alyssa lying in her coffin when given the choice, and I had not ever seen a dead person until my early forties. Most of us have never seen death up close, or if we have, it may be limited to only a few times in the thick cloud of emotion. Many people have been to open-casket funerals for a relative or friend, but the body they see has been made up to look serene and sleepy, as if at any moment the deceased may wake up and climb out of the casket in his or her Sunday best. And the fear that accompanies the visual of death creates another layer of fear to overcome when contemplating our own mortality. We know we should be there when someone we love dies, if we can, but we often can't bear the thought of occupying the same space as someone who passes on from this world because we are watching a preview of our own future. Looking carefully at the moments just before and after death and what happens to the body can help ease us into that sacred space when life is tottering and death is calling.

The spiritual Buddhist master Sogyal Rinpoche wrote a guide to help people of the West handle death in the spiritual way that he observes in his own Eastern traditions, traditions that he finds lacking in the West. Sogyal Rinpoche runs a network of Buddhist centers in dozens of countries around the world called Rigpa, which means "intelligence" or "awareness." He believes that we have to help the dying dwell on what they have accomplished in this life and what they can feel proud of so that they can spend their last hours concentrating on their virtues and leave this world on the journey to the next in greater peace. He notes that people who are dying are "frequently extremely vulnerable to guilt, regret, and depression";[2] and that while it is important to listen to their fears and disappointments, it is also crucial that we help them see the goodness within. In addition, Rinpoche recommends that those present with the dying be scrupulous in their emotional control for the dying person's sake:

> I advise everyone to do their best to work out attachment and grief with the dying person before death comes: Cry together, express your love, and say goodbye, but try to finish with this process before the actual moment of death arrives. If possible, it is best if friends and relatives do not show excessive grief at the moment of death, because the consciousness of the dying person is at that moment exceptionally vulnerable. The *Tibetan Book of the Dead* says that your crying and tears around a person's bedside are experienced like thunder and hail.[3]

The idea of allowing the dying the space to lessen their attachments to the living may seem counterintuitive to those raised in the West, where the moment right before death is the time we all crowd the person dying and wail. In the original *Tibetan Book of the Dead*, Padmasambhava shares his thoughts:

> *Now when the cycle of dying dawns upon me,*
> *I will abandon all grasping, yearning, and attachment,*
> *Enter undistracted into clear awareness of the teaching. . . .*
> *As I leave this compound body of flesh and blood*
> *I will know it to be a transitory illusion.*

Unlike the belief that nothing is more real than being present as someone passes on, the Buddhist tradition believes that mortal death is an illusion since it is just the beginning of rebirth. To prepare for rebirth, the soul must lack attachments to people, things and the past. In contrast to ancient Egyptians, who kept their prized possessions in preparation for the next life, Buddhist preparation involves detachment from all things and people.

Looking at different faiths at the moment of death takes us far afield from Far Eastern death scenes. For centuries, people died at home in their beds. Doctors and nurses visited them and provided bedside care in the presence of family, friends and the comfort of a favorite pillow and familiar furnishings. Clergy spent decades ministering to patients and participating in the family milestones, helping to create the spiritual framework to face death. That intimacy eased the journey from a place of the known to a place of the unknown.

In the middle of the last century, this image of death at home gave way to death in a hospital setting, a cold and sterile place where each person loses the individuality of clothing, furnishings and private space. Now death is not the only unknown; everything else is unfamiliar as well. There is no soft pillow and no intimacy. There is only sterility. We whisk away the sick and dying to another place, an impersonal building, usually of mammoth proportions painted in pale gray, nondescript beige or sickly green that reeks of illness. The dying are served bland food in plastic containers on cafeteria trays, with none of the nurturing touches of the home kitchen. The enduring compassion we have for the dying when they live and die among us is replaced by distant caring, by remote feelings that dissipate when we are no longer in the presence of the sick.

If you are dying, instead of your personal physician visiting you at home, you will most likely be taken care of by a doctor who shoulders the burden of hundreds of patients in a clinic or hospital and a nursing staff beset by heavy demands. You are known to most of the medical staff by the white board on your door and the chart on your bed: the pancreatic cancer in room 545. You have lost your self to the impersonality of disease. The presence of your family and friends is limited to visiting hours determined by someone else. You are surrounded by machines that have the capacity to prolong your breathing and your heartbeat but will, in most cases, never bring you back to the life you once enjoyed. The anesthetized atmosphere robs you of your dignity and your most basic sense of personhood.

Of course, we should be cared for in places where our medical needs can be most professionally addressed. Doctors and nurses cannot be faulted for trying to see as many people as they can within a reasonable time period. They are doing their jobs. A little tenderness would be nice, but the fault does not lie with the staff. It lies with the system we have created to manage death, one that tangles us in complicated insurance processes, difficult "do not resuscitate" decisions and confusing medical jargon. Once the process of death sets in and is only days, weeks or months away, some of our fixed notions of hospital deaths should be challenged by a gentler, kinder way to leave this earth: in the bosom of love and family and surroundings that make us feel most reassured that life will go on, even if our own life will not continue. The hospice system has challenged the sterility of death, but hospice care is still not the norm for most of the world's dying.

Those who have little contact with death know little about the rituals attendant upon the dead body in their own culture or faith, let alone the faiths or cultures of others. Little in our lives occasions familiarity with such details. Even if we have been with someone at the moment of death, we have little understanding of the physiology of the dead and what awaits them in the days before burial or cremation. We've heard of death rattles and rigor mortis, but we usually associate death creepiness with second-rate horror films. We know about death from movies, where starlets close their eyes, heavy with mascara, and sleep forever, and we hope that when our time comes, it's Hollywood-style and peaceful.

The psychiatrist Vivian Rakoff writes that "mourning is essentially a process of unlearning the expected presence of the deceased."[4] Nowhere is this more prominent than in the first hours after death. There is the unlearning of presence and the learning of a new vocabulary around loss. No one knows quite what to do, whom to call, how to make the arrangements, particularly if the deceased had no requests or was not part of a religious community where members face major life events with regulated, anticipated practices, almost like being on ritual cruise control.

The first moments after death challenge us with their linguistic nuances. If you're not used to the change of language that death necessitates, each admission of the death becomes another visit with pain. "She's gone." "What would he do now?" "Where did she put that?" Unlearning the presence of the dead is a complex process that begins with shock and reverberates for the days, weeks and years following the death. Years after her father died, a friend said she had just returned from visiting her parents: "I didn't mean that. I meant my mother. Not my parents." She stumbled and was flustered as if trying to understand what occasioned her mistake instead of appreciating that decades of having two parents could not be unraveled in the short span of 36 months.

The presence of the immediately deceased, however, brooks no mistakes and makes us aware of the finality of life especially at this liminal time, after death and before burial. Liminal times—the in-between transitions we experience—are usually crowded with religious ritual. People in faith communities usually benefit from assigned, expected structures and behaviors that slide them into ambiguities with a life vest. Rituals pillow our anxieties and provide a buffer of familiarity when confronting the strange newness of situations we've never been in before.

Take, for example, the intricate rituals involved in preparing the body for burial in the ancient Japanese tradition of encoffinment. The ritual is masterfully depicted in Yojiro Takita's film *Departures*. Takita spent ten years observing this ritual, performed mostly in rural areas of Japan, and he based the movie, in part, on the book *Coffinman: The Journal of a Buddhist Mortician*, by Aoki Shinmon. Most Japanese follow Buddhist burial traditions of cremation that are hundreds of years old. In the early days of the Buddhist incursion into Japan, only monks and religious dignitaries were cremated because of the expense of wood to make the fires. Over time the practice spread, and now nearly a hundred percent of Japanese people undergo cremation at death. The night before and the day of the funeral, a wake is conducted, where friends and family stay with the body all night. This is loosely based on Jodo Buddhist practices, where students of the Buddha stayed up all night learning his teachings in front of his body.

The film has at its center a young cellist looking for a job after his orchestra dissolves. He answers an ad in the paper for a high-paying job involving "departures" and believes it is for a travel agency. At the interview he finds out that there was a mistake in the ad, and it is really for a job involving the "departed." He is to assist the undertaker in encoffinment, doing the elaborate washing and makeup ceremony of the Japanese and placing the body in a coffin before cremation. The secretary at the company shows him the coffin display in the office and the range of prices but shrugs after showing him the most expensive, carved cypress wood coffin: "They all burn the same way." While this may be true, the person preparing the bodies and the makeup tries to make departed loved ones look their personal best. The family kneels in front of the body at a slight distance to watch the preparation, although they are not allowed to see any skin except the face.

The young cellist, who at first is horrified by this job prospect, changes his tune as he watches his boss gently and lovingly place the hands of the deceased together around a set of pearls, cross the feet, dress the body and then invite the family to wipe the face of the departed with a white cloth, a symbolic gesture signifying the first bath the body will take in the next world. The family moistens the lips of the deceased, a ritual called "water of the last moment." The turning point for the cellist comes when he and the mortician are leaving the home of a devastated family after the ritual dressing ceremony. A bereaved husband runs after them to say, "She never looked so beautiful." The cellist realizes then that the gift to the family is not just in making the body look serene and peaceful as it exits this world, but in the tenderness of the mortician's touch as he dignifies the last moments of the deceased person's presence among the living.

• • •

In many religions, the dead body is treated as a sacred object that must be gently and thoughtfully cleaned and prepared for burial. Often it is through the treatment of the dead body that we begin to understand the central tenets of any particular faith. I learned that through speaking with Fadwa and Cheryl, two women—one Muslim and the other Jewish—who are both devoted to their respective ancient rituals of handling bodies of loved ones immediately after death.

Fadwa came to the United States in 1993 from Sur Baher, a small village in Israel between Jerusalem and Bethlehem. She settled in Trenton, New Jersey, where she lives in a small house with her husband and two daughters. When her husband died, her stepsons helped take care of her. Her mother was in the process of dying when we spoke, and now she would pay the care forward.

Fadwa has a big laugh and a happy, round face enhanced by the tight *hijab* she wears on her head. The night we spoke, her hair was tucked into a black headpiece that striped her forehead and a flowing beige *hijab* that folded onto her shoulders. She wore a long black robe, an *abaya*, over her clothes. This one was plain black polyester with lavender and gold detailing down the sleeve and an intricate pattern in the front. Very expensive *abayas* generally come from Dubai and can cost hundreds of dollars. These are usually worn on holidays and festive occasions. But Fadwa confessed that, being a widow, she did not have the money to indulge in such purchases, although sometimes she spoiled her daughters.

Muslim school is ten thousand dollars a year, far too much for a widow supported by her stepsons, so Fadwa's daughters go to public school and have separate instruction in their faith a few times a week after school. Fadwa herself teaches such classes in her home to five- and six-year-olds. She knows that her oldest daughter stands out as a

Muslim in public school, but she isn't disturbed by this. School in America is a melting pot for children of many different races and religions. She sees this as a place of great opportunity for her daughters. Fadwa is very grateful for the tolerance and opportunities she finds in American life but holds on tightly to traditions that ground her in the chaos of modernity. Fadwa brought me into her life so I could understand death within a rich context of traditions and rituals. Death was not separate from tradition but a continuation of it. As she spoke, I saw the depth of her compassion and the network of community and friendships that anchor her life.

Fadwa's husband had been previously married, as had she. She only went to school until the ninth grade; although she liked to learn, no one pushed her. It was uncommon in her village for Muslim women to advance to higher education, although she spoke insistently about her daughters going to college and having the education she did not. She married for the first time at eighteen and spent the intervening years between ninth grade and her wedding learning to cook and make a home. She describes how she met her husband and how most traditional Muslims meet each other. A man sees a woman or is told about a woman who may be a good match. He then goes to her house or family to inquire about her. Her family then inquires about him. If both sides seem religiously and financially compatible, the families get together. "Then you bring the coffee." Fadwa said this as if I would instantly recognize the significance.

"What do you mean?" I ask.

"You know, you bring out the coffee on a tray. He sees you and you see him, and he decides if he likes you and you like him." The future of a life together is decided over a caffeinated beverage. This could give Starbucks a whole new side industry: matchmaking.

Fadwa's first marriage lasted only nine years because her husband couldn't have children, and his family was not nice to her. She could have put up with her childlessness but not their meanness. Her second husband, also snagged over coffee, already had five children of his own. He was also a diabetic, a health detail not revealed during the coffee ritual or at all before the marriage. Fadwa had two daughters with him but soon found herself taking care of a very sick man. For nine years she looked after him: sat by his hospital bed, lifted him into his wheelchair and, finally, closed his eyelids in the middle of the night when he died. Closing the eyelids of the dead is an important ritual in Islam because Umm Salama, one of Mohammed's wives, closed his eyelids after he died.

Muslims are entreated to be kind and patient in the company of the dying and to induce the dying to pray for forgiveness. They traditionally recite verses from the Koran and also encourage the one dying to say prayers to Allah so that the last words on one's lips are words of devotion and faith: "I bear witness that there is no God but Allah."

When the dying depart from this world, they are covered in a clean sheet. Preparations for the burial begin immediately. Relatives and friends are discouraged from excessive grieving based on the experience that Mohammed had when he lost his own son: "The eyes shed tears and the heart is grieved, but we will not say anything except which pleases our Lord." It is fundamental to Islam to accept the fate that Allah has determined.

Before prayer, Muslims do the *wudhu*, the ritualistic wash of the entire body, making sure that their clothing is also clean. Ablutions are very important in the Islamic tradition. The Koran says that "Allah loves those who turn to Him constantly, and He loves those who keep themselves pure and clean." Mohammed once said that "Cleanliness is half of faith." Muslims make sure they are ritually clean before touching a Koran. Purifying both the body and one's clothing is called *tahara*; the exact same word is used in Hebrew.

The details of daily Muslim observance in washing and prayer that Fadwa shares are reflective of Islamic death rituals. Prayer, washing and body covering are all central to the way the Muslim body is treated after death. Men and women are separated in most strictly observant Muslim societies, and this is no different at the time of death. If a woman dies, then another woman gives her the *wudhu*, the ritual bathing of her hands, her face, her head, her ears, her chest, her neck and finally her legs. Two to three women are involved in the process because the body has to be moved, and this can be physically strenuous. The woman who is assigned the actual washing is usually someone trustworthy and close to the person who died. Fadwa has bathed several relatives and friends. Her own elderly mother was in a coma when we spoke, and I asked Fadwa if she would give her mother the *wudhu* or if it was awkward. "Of course. It is my honor." Fadwa was not complacent about death but not afraid of it either. Having taken care of a dying husband, Fadwa saw death as an occasional visitor in her life and not one she was going to turn away at the door.

When Muslims write their wills, they can pick the person who will give them the *wudhu* because it is such an honor. The *wudhu* is not time-consuming; it only takes five minutes, and then the body is taken off the table for dressing in the *kafn*. The *kafn* is a long, white, inexpensive cloth bought in a specialty store that has an opening for the head and loosely worn pants. The *kafn* is wrapped around the body, covering every body surface but the face. The cloth is wrapped, and a long tail is left at the head and feet that is later bunched together. Only the face is visible. The garment must lie loosely on the body—never sewn—so that the soul will be able to leave the body comfortably on the Day of Judgment. The same ritual is performed regardless of gender.

After the *wudhu* and wrapping in the *kafn*, the body is placed in a central room in the house so that relatives can pay their last respects;

they often kiss the person goodbye, usually on the forehead. After the farewell, the white tails of the *kafn* around the head and legs are tied, and the body is covered in a blanket and taken to the local mosque. In the United States, the body must be moved in a casket. "But in my country, we do not place bodies in a box," Fadwa said. "We just cover them in a sheet." This, interestingly, is the custom among both Jews and Muslims in Israel: dead bodies are covered with cloth and not boxed as eulogies are recited. There is something more raw and graphic to this practice. It brings participants closer to the experience of death by not hiding the body in a casket but allowing for the draped form of the deceased to lie in covered profile. It can be quite disturbing for those who have never seen it before. My first time witnessing it threw me into a flurry of anxiety: the way the cloth draped the profile of the head, accentuating the peak of the nose, and then the slope down the chest forced the admission of loss in a way that a rectangular casket could not. The body is then transported to the cemetery.

At the cemetery, those designated the honor of carrying the body or coffin stand on both sides of a gurney and pray the *salat-al-janazah*, prayers for the dead for atonement and a good passage into the next world. The imam stands by himself in front of the group and faces Mecca. With focused intent, the imam leads the group in prayer or *du'a* for the deceased, following the words of Mohammed:

O God, forgive our living and our dead, those who are present among us and those who are absent, our young and our old, our males and our females. O God, whomever You keep alive, keep him alive in Islam, and whoever You cause to die, cause him to die with faith. O God, do not deprive us of the reward and do not cause us to go astray after this. O God, forgive him and have mercy on him, keep him safe and sound and forgive him, honor his rest and ease his entrance; wash him with water and snow and hail, and cleanse him of sin as a white garment is cleansed of dirt. O God, give him a home better than his home and a family better than his family. O God, admit him to Paradise and protect him from the torment of the grave and the torment of Hell-fire; make his grave spacious and fill it with light.

The funeral prayers use many names of God that are excerpted from the Koran and dedicated to the dead. Gender differences are apparent now. The *janazah* prayers are only performed by men; women are not allowed to go to the cemetery. The men bury the body, cover it with earth, read the Koran and ask God to help the deceased. Traditional Muslims believe that once the body is in the grave, two angels come and question the deceased, and then the soul ascends into the sky with the angels.

I wondered about this angel-led interrogation process. What sort of questions do you get asked at this point, and how do your answers determine what happens next? In the Talmud, there is a famous passage that states that when you get to *Shamayim*, heaven, God asks the newly departed soul some questions about the worthiness of its owner's past life: (1) Did you deal honestly in business? (2) Did you make time to study? (3) Did you have and raise children? (4) Did you work on behalf of the world's redemption?[5] (5) Did you engage in wisdom? (6) Did you learn one thing from another? Remember: this is heaven. You're not supposed to lie.

Fadwa then lets me in on a little secret. *Shahada*, she tells me, is special. In other words, jihadists, those who die fulfilling a holy mission that involves martyrdom, get special treatment when it comes to the rituals of the dead. No angels question them, nor do they have the *wudhu* or the *kafn*. When it comes to jihadists you don't wash the body or the clothes; they are buried with the blood on them. I didn't know if this is because of shame or because of pride, and I did not want to insult Fadwa by asking.

Muslims are discouraged from making elaborate and expensive grave markers. Humility is key in these rituals. The dead are often visited on holidays, but the site is not to become a place of excessive mourning. Fadwa tells me that Muslims are not supposed to pull out their hair or rip their clothes and scream, much as you might want to when you lose someone you love.

There is a brief mourning period, three days, usually in the home of the deceased. Fadwa tells me that visitors bring food because mourners are not supposed to cook their own meals. The mourners give visitors black coffee and dates. Men and women often visit at separate times and always sit separately during the condolence period. Widows mourn longer: four months and ten days. The widow must stay at home and not adorn herself. She also cannot remarry during this time.

The burial process is sacred in Muslim tradition because this is an important time of reckoning and judgment for the deceased. Muslims believe in heaven and hell. On Judgment Day you will be responsible for your past, and you can even be punished in the grave. Fadwa trembles a little when she says this; it frightens her. Mohammed said that three things outlive you when you die: the charity you gave; the knowledge you disseminated that will live beyond you, and the children who live after you and pray on your behalf. Fadwa prays for her sick mother and gives charity in the hope that she will die peacefully. "I worry about my mom, but I need her to be comfortable. Her body is shutting down. When you look at her, you can see she is in pain, and then I am in pain. God makes some lives easy. God makes some lives hard."


Cheryl would probably say the same thing. Within the Jewish tradition, dead bodies undergo a process called *tahara*, ritual purification, generally within twelve to twenty-four hours after death. These purifications are performed by members of a small, often quite secretive volunteer society called the *chevra kadisha,* literally a "sacred society" or group. Cheryl is a registered nurse and lactation consultant by profession. She has been doing *taharot* (the plural of the word) for twenty-one years in Kansas City. She is in her early fifties, beautifully dressed, with the kind of smooth skin women have in fashion magazines. I wondered how she got started in the business of death. It seemed like an odd volunteer cause, especially for an attractive and busy professional. She told me that she started when she was becoming more Jewishly observant and had recently switched her children into a parochial school. She heard that a third person was needed to do a *tahara.* Kansas has a small Jewish community, she explained, so people can't really bow out of responsibilities. In fact, the school her children attended offered tuition breaks in exchange for communal service to incentivize people to volunteer, especially for the tough jobs.

The process of *tahara* is complex and involves a lot of moving parts for someone who is not moving. When a Jewish person who requests a traditional burial dies, the funeral home calls someone on the *chevra kadisha* staff, all of whom are volunteers. As in Muslim tradition, men wash men and women wash women. Three to five people are invited to participate at a time, depending on who is available and the size of the body. That many people are necessary because the body must be moved and washed while the appropriate prayers are recited. Water must be poured almost continually on the body. It is physical work and too much for one person to handle alone. Cheryl shared the moment of initial anxiety when the phone rings: "When you see the number come in on caller ID, for a split second you feel like you don't want to pick up the phone, but then you pick it up, and you're grateful for the opportunity to do it."

Generally, the *tahara* is done the morning of the funeral, but the ritual is also performed the night before the burial, usually but not always at the funeral home. The room has a table where the body has been placed and houses the casket where the body will be gently deposited after the purification ritual is completed. The participants wear surgical gowns, waterproof shoes, masks and gloves to protect against any disease that the body may have carried, since none of the volunteers are privy to information about the dead person. Cheryl said that in the *taharot* she's participated in, the women take a moment to center themselves and get in the right frame of mind. "You can't just go from the carpool lane to a *tahara*." The women usually say some variation of a personal prayer: "Let us take a moment to reflect on the work we are about to do. Let us act with humility and treat this person with dignity and respect." It helps, she said, if she can think of the person as a mother, an aunt, or a friend so that she can invest the lifting and washing with a sense of love. I asked Cheryl if she ever did a *tahara* on an actual relative. Her eyes lit up: "I did it for my own grandmother. Some rabbis don't allow you to do that for a family member. But I felt that I sent her off. I was the last goodbye. I loved her so much. I sent her off with so much love. I really did."

The first washing begins with warm water, and Cheryl describes it as if she were washing a child. Anything foreign or external to the body must be removed: nail polish, the gum of IV tape, dirt. The hair is usually washed. The body is covered at all times with a sheet, and the volunteers only see the part of the body they are washing at any particular moment. One person says a blessing and recites psalms as the others lift the body and wash it. Cheryl describes it as an inclusive practice, because anyone who wants to participate can. Even if they don't have the physical strength to work with the body, they are able to offer prayers. In larger communities, there is usually a *mikveh* or ritual bath in the funeral home, and the body is hoisted in a harness into the water and fully immersed. When no *mikveh* is available, the women wash their hands to purify them and then take three buckets of tap water that has been mixed with pure rainwater, which is poured over the entire body, with the sheet removed. The holy water must touch every part of the body: the ears, the back, the hair; it must come in contact with every orifice. Then the women in unison say the Hebrew words *"Tahara he"* three times, which means "She is pure." If the body soils itself in the process, which often happens, or a foreign mark is later discovered, then the whole process must be repeated. It is a very meticulous ritual.

The body is then dried and dressed in simple white cotton shrouds that are called *tachrichim* in Hebrew. The shrouds consist of a number of pieces that generally mimic the clothing worn by the high priest in the Temple, as described in the book of Leviticus, chapter 28. The shrouds divide the upper and lower body; there is a shirt and a pair of trousers closed at the feet. Once dressed, the body is placed in a simple wooden casket. As mentioned earlier, the dead should be buried in simple white shrouds and a simple wooden casket to equalize the experience of death throughout the community. Death is not to be marked with any measures of status, just as the experience of death is the great equalizer of the human condition.

The very last ritual before burial demands that the volunteers place soil of Jerusalem on the eyes, heart and genitals. Cheryl explains that these body parts are most associated with sin; they are what can draw you away from God and from others, so the last step of purification is to sanctify them and connect the person to the holiest of places. Judaism is fundamentally about sanctifying time and space, and at this very holy time in the cycle of the body, these particles from holy places are used to elevate the body. The cover is then placed on the casket, and then the casket is moved out of the room, making sure that the deceased's feet are facing the exit. The entire process takes about an hour and a half.

Cheryl shared her most profound experience of *tahara* with me in a slow, almost mournful way. It was a Friday morning, and she had taken a young woman to the *mikveh* for the traditional immersion brides undergo right before a wedding. She then went straight to the local funeral home to perform a *tahara* for a woman who died of anorexia. Later in the day, she went to the hospital to assist a new mother struggling to nurse her infant. She knew all three women personally. They were all twenty-five years old.

She finds that the hardest purifications are those she does for Holocaust survivors. I assumed that it was hard for Cheryl because each death amplifies the loss of that generation, the loss of another witness to history. That was true, she said, but there was more to it. "We remove everything that is not natural to the body, but you can't wash off the numbers that are tattooed on an Auschwitz survivor's arm."

But then Cheryl smiled when she spoke of Molly. On Fridays, Cheryl always gets a manicure, and one Friday afternoon, after she had just finished a *tahara*, she found herself in the salon sitting next to Molly, a woman who was suffering from late-stage ovarian cancer. Molly was always beautifully coifed. Cheryl told the manicurist where she had just come from and Molly, overhearing the conversation, told Cheryl that she wanted to be cremated. Cheryl asked her why she would want to do that to her body, pointing out that Molly obviously nurtured her body very carefully in this life. Molly was adamant; when they were done, they said their goodbyes. Three months later, Cheryl got a call from the funeral home to do a *tahara*. Molly had died. "One of the people in the *chevra* said that she changed her mind. The daughter called and was so grateful that she and her father could visit her gravesite. Everyone else in the family had been cremated."

I asked Cheryl if there were any unusual requests. She once had a woman who insisted on being buried in a St. John's knit suit. The woman said she would not have a *tahara* unless she was able to spend her eternal life in this outfit. "Under the circumstances we let it go."

And though she's bathed a child who was buried with a favorite teddy bear, she discourages families against veering from tradition. It's the simplicity and humility of death that brings people together. We're all the same when we go.


Cheryl's first *tahara* was done out of obligation, but hundreds and hundreds of *taharot* later, she speaks about the process as one of the most spiritually moving practices she observes. After her initial experience with *tahara*, Cheryl learned that the people who performed this *mitzvah*, or "commandment," were a tight-knit group, in her case, of older women. She describes the society as an extraordinary collection of people who come to the ritual with a sense of intentionality and personal maturity and who grow spiritually through the observance of this commandment. A woman writing about her experience after finishing a *tahara* shared how intimate and different everything suddenly looked and felt: "Returning home that evening I was struck by an intense awareness of my husband's warm body close to mine as we went to sleep. I listened to his heartbeat and the rush of blood running through his body."[6] The sense of the physical self becomes highly pronounced, about oneself and others. A man described how in tune he was with the presence of another body while he performed this ritual: "When I look at the deceased, I can perceive pain and despair, especially if there are obvious signs, such as bedsores or missing limbs. I feel that I am enabling the soul to pass through a veil, leaving behind it all the sorrow and suffering of his final days."[7]

That feeling is often professed by many who perform this commandment. They leave this experience a little pummeled, with more patience for the irritations of everyday life and other people. Cheryl told me that although the room where the *tahara* is performed is almost never dark, she is very aware when she finishes of the bright light outside, and a deep need to breathe slowly and loudly, feeling very blessed to be among the living. The transition from the sphere of death back into life is not made smoothly.

Rabbi Irving Greenberg writes powerfully of the importance of the rituals that take place right after death: "Death appears to be the ultimate state of being cut off and isolated. But love responds by stepping forward, in solidarity, to be with the deceased. This treatment is irrefutable testimony that this departed one was and is bound up in the bonds of life and love."[8] These rituals confirm that the body is sanctified, even when it is not animated. It housed the soul for the duration of time that a human being "lived" in it. The act lets the family and all other mourners know that the cessation of bodily functions does not mean that the body should be treated with any less dignity or sanctity. Quite the opposite: once the body dies and the one who "occupied" it for a lifetime is no longer present, the community of family and friends becomes its steward.

Cheryl's work as a lactation consultant allows her to spend a lot of time on the other side of the human timeline as well. It was easy enough to see the appeal of helping new mothers nurse their babies, but why was she so drawn to the loss of selfhood?

In the Jewish tradition, we believe that the soul hovers over the body, and I really believe that. I feel that there is an aura in the room and that this body is a shell, and the soul is no longer in the body. But you know that it is not completely over because the soul has a hard time detaching itself from the body. It's been there for a whole lifetime. You're ushering this person from this world to the next world. No one else can see the body after the *tahara*. It's just an incredible privilege to be there.

Cheryl lost her own son, who was in his twenties, to suicide about a year before our conversation. Since he died, she has not been able to do a *tahara*. It's all a little too close for comfort, she said, too raw to be that close to death. But when I asked her about what she gets out of her experience with the *chevra kadisha*, she nods thoughtfully and speaks softly.

> Every single time I do it, I get something different. You're never look-
> ing at the body. You're working on a vessel of God, and you feel that
> when you're with the body. I actually know a lot of the people I work
> on because it's a small community. I thought it would make me anx-
> ious, but it is actually very comforting because you're in the presence
> of something very godly. I'm touched every time I do a *tahara*. I'm
> constantly aware of how fragile life really is.

Cheryl described the moment she finishes a *tahara* with much the same attachment: "You come out of there, and you breathe the fresh air, even though there's no odor and there's ventilation. It still takes your breath away. And when you walk out I always take a deep breath just feeling that life. There's nothing like it."

I wanted to understand that universe of grace that Fadwa and Cheryl had created, the way they make the final passage so dignified and holy. I called Rachel, a young mother in my own community, to ask her if I could attend a *tahara* with her. I was nervous about it, having only seen one dead person in my whole life. Seeing and handling a dead person was a difference of nontraversable magnitude in my mind. But here was this woman, years younger than I, who was a team leader of the *chevra kadisha*. And she had been doing ritual washings for over twenty years.

"We start young in my family," Rachel said.

"How young?"

"I did my first *tahara* at thirteen."

"Thirteen?" She had been confronting her mortality from the age when I was going to dorky bar mitzvah parties and talking about clothes and braces. This just confirmed my belief that people who engage in these acts of goodness are wrapped in a cloud of extraordinariness.

Rachel explained her early start. Her mother has been the head of the *chevra kadisha* for decades and had taught her children not to fear death. When Rachel was thirteen, a few people she knew had suffered terrible deaths, and she begged her mother to go to a *tahara* as a way of dealing with her own pain. Since then, she has helped train many other women, inducting them into the commandment. She described bathing her first suicide, a woman with rope burns around her neck. She told me that she has asked her mother to accompany her on certain occasions when the body has been maimed or defaced through violence. Rachel's mother taught her that everyone deserves to die *b'kavod*, the Hebrew word for "with honor." "I used to be afraid to look," Rachel said. "But because of her I can." I knew that Rachel would help me open my eyes. I sensed it. She told me that she would call me when the time came.

The time, however, was not coming. Since you can get a call at any time, I had to leave my schedule wide open. This was not an easy feat. Wednesday night passed and then Thursday night. No call. I made sure that Saturday night was free. Rachel assured me that a lot of people die over the weekend. A friend asked if we wanted to go to the movies. "I can't. I have other plans." I didn't explain. But Saturday, Sunday and Monday night passed. No call. Just my luck. When I had finally readied myself to wash a dead person, everyone decided to stay alive. I was reminded of the medieval Hebrew poet Abraham Ibn Ezra, who believed he was born under a bad star. In one poem, he writes:

*If I sold shrouds,*
*No one would die.*
*If I sold lamps,*
*Then, in the sky,*
*The sun, for spite,*
*Would shine by night.*

Maybe I should take up poetry while I wait.

I have just returned home from my first *tahara*. My stomach is in knots. A slight acidic taste chokes my throat, as if I am about to throw up but not quite. My mouth is incredibly dry.

A week and a bit after I made my request, Rachel sent me a text: Thursday night. I met her at seven o'clock at her house. When I showed up, she looked at me, and the first thing she said was, "Where are your boots?" She was wearing Wellingtons. I had never asked about the dress code.

We picked up the other women on the team and headed out to the funeral home. It is located on a main thoroughfare, sandwiched between a luxury car dealership and a cheap furniture store. The *tahara* room is in the basement. It felt dark and creepy to be there. When Rachel opened the combination lock, I took in the signs on the wall about biohazardous waste and the one bold poster that said, "Take pride in your work." It seemed so out of place and yet so appropriate to the task. I was stunningly conscious of my surroundings. When we got down the stairs, Rachel checked the room and said that the body had not been deposited on the table. "Erica, let's get the body."

Wait: did she say my name? Yes. She said my name. Did she say "Erica, let's get the body"? Yes she did.

Rachel threw me into it the way that a parent throws a child into a swimming pool, with no time to take note of my fear. We entered a large room with shelves of caskets and opened the locked door of the freezer. There were two wooden caskets with documentation tucked on top and one body on a metal gurney covered in a sheet. It must be her.

The woman was in her eighties. Rachel had told us on the car journey that she has edemas, swellings on her body that we may notice but that are nothing medically unusual. I pushed the gurney at the head, and we gathered into the green-tiled room where the *tahara* was to take place. Rachel guided us through the steps. Surprisingly, at forty-five, I was the oldest woman on the team. The youngest was Rachel's niece, a senior in college. She has been doing *taharot* for two and a half years.

Rachel unzipped the body bag while it was on the gurney and close to the table in the washing room. We rolled its white plastic sheeting underneath the woman and gently removed it, and a white cotton sheet was placed over her. Underneath the sheet, I saw tufts of gray and white hair sticking out from the form of her head. Rachel asked me to cradle her head as we moved her onto the metal table in the center of the room. As we moved her and dressed her, holding her head—the holiest part of the body in Jewish tradition—made me feel like I was embracing a living, thinking, loving being, although all her functioning had stopped. I was reminded of a nurse I spoke to who said that she saw her first dead body at eighteen. It was a young man who was brought into the ER after a car accident; he was dead, but the watch on his wrist kept ticking. She couldn't stop thinking about that ticking watch and how time continued even when his own time had stopped.

I was standing beside Rachel on the left side of the body, and the other three women stood on the other side of the table. When we leaned the body over to one side, Rachel called on me to bring wet paper towels. She cleaned the body carefully, and for a long time the body continued to release fluids and matter from its orifices. This was a rather shocking introduction to the holiness of this commandment. I wasn't quite prepared. I looked away.

We are so consciously aware of our own bodily fluids and emissions, but to see those of another human being—even those of a dead stranger—felt like a betrayal of intimacy. And it made me appreciate how intricate the rituals around burial are in every faith because we never want the body to become profane in our minds and then somehow become disposable. If we don't treat the body with the utmost tenderness and sanctity, we betray our uniqueness. We become a hodgepodge of skin and organs and cells without the animation of a soul and a mind and a spirit. Later, when I cleaned the woman's body, I noticed how cold and rigid it was. It felt like a person but not like a person. But still a person.

After cleaning the body thoroughly and removing any external particles like medical tape, powder and lotion, we removed our surgical gowns and gloves and did another washing of our hands. Then we prepared for the ritual washing. Most funeral homes do not have a ritual bath in which to immerse the dead body. We took three buckets of cold water to simulate a *mikveh* and immersed the straps on the side of gurney into the water to purify them symbolically. We then strapped the woman in and tilted the gurney from head to toe, pouring three buckets of water over her body so that it could sluice over her and the metal table. Now I understood about the boots. Boots would have been useful.

Slowly we dressed this woman in white garments, covering the face first and then the feet and legs. I helped Rachel tie the pants; the ties were swirled seven times, reflecting the number of days of creation, symbolizing completion and perfection in Jewish law. Then Rachel tied them into the three loops of the Hebrew letter *shin*, which represents the name of God the protector. This was the sign this woman would take with her into the ground. We put a loose shirt on her and then another jacket. This woman, whose whole life was now reduced to flesh on a stainless-steel plate, was now covered in white cotton.

Rachel asked two women to bring in the wooden coffin that was lined in straw. We raised the gurney and then all of us lifted the woman slowly and methodically into the coffin. This time, I was in charge of her feet. Rachel lifted the face veil and put pottery shards on her eyes and elsewhere and then dirt from Jerusalem's Mount of Olives, just as Cheryl had said. Talking is only permitted when it relates to the ritual washing process; I asked Rachel about the shards and she said that we are all broken vessels and that is how we live and die. She asked another woman and myself to get the cover of the coffin, with the Star of David three-quarters of the way down, from the other room. I took the side that said "FEET," and we gently fit it on top of the coffin. Rachel had us all surround the coffin and then she closed her eyes and asked *mechila*, "forgiveness," from the deceased if we had not treated her body with the utmost respect. As she said this, I felt myself trembling, my eyes welling with tears. I was dumbstruck by the request for forgiveness from someone who could not answer, simply to pardon us if we had mishandled her. Rachel ended by saying, "Go in peace." Her niece said the same. They have been trained well.

It was a humbling evening, a holy evening. On the way home the woman in the front passenger seat turned to me and said, "Erica, you'd never guess that this was your first time." And I was shocked because I thought my skin must have been visibly green. I tried to suppress the acidic taste in my throat. The small car brought the five of us physically even closer. I did not know any of these women well but had you told me that any one of them would wash my body when my time came, I would have said, "Thank God. Go in peace." When

Rachel dropped me off I thanked her and said, "Call me again if you need me."

The Buddhist, Muslim and Jewish approaches to the immediately deceased stand in sharp contrast to two other ways we treat the body at death: embalming and cremation. Embalming is an extremely old practice popularized by the ancient Egyptians but also used by the Incas, the Chinese and other ancient peoples to extend the "life" of the body and protect it from initial decomposition. The soul is ostensibly still housed in a preserved corpse. Embalming is not only viewed as a spiritual tradition in some religions but often a practical measure if the deceased needed to be moved from one place to another distant location for burial. Embalming was used often during the American Civil War and for military purposes to rejoin dead soldiers with their families after a significant passage of time.

Among morticians, embalming increased in popularity with the discovery of formaldehyde in the nineteenth century, which was less toxic (to the mortician) than the arsenic used before. Embalming is used today not only to preserve the body but also to help the cadaver look more lifelike for viewing, especially if the burial is days or weeks away from the actual death. The body is placed on a table with private parts covered for modesty. Dead people usually don't embarrass easily, but these sentiments, like so many in the ritual bathings described earlier, preserve the dignity of the body for those who take care of it after death. It is then washed with disinfectant. The lips are often sewn or glued together. The face is supposed to look relaxed. Embalming chemicals are injected into the blood vessels with a centrifugal pump while the body is massaged to make sure that the fluid is evenly distributed. A small cut is made just above the navel, and a trocar is placed in the body to drain or aspirate the internal body fluids and replace them with embalming chemicals. A trocar is not a friendly funeral tool. It is a sharp, pointed surgical instrument fitted with a small tube called a cannula that gets inserted into a body cavity and is used for drainage. It is thrust into the sternum, turned spirally, and pulled in and out of the abdomen or chest cavity. The incision is then sutured together. The rest of the embalming is usually done eight to ten hours later, when the skin tissue is more firm and dry. The entire process takes several hours. The embalmer's goal is to make the body look as close to living as possible. But if you read "amusing" accounts of the mortuary business—*Mortuary Confidential, Down Among the Dead Men,* or *Curtains*—you encounter all kinds of mishaps: wrong stabs and overenthusiastic cutters whose path to body restoration is strewn with mistakes. These accounts make for unusual, if not uncomfortable, entertainment, as long as you pretend you're reading fiction.

Then there's cremation as a way of handling the dead. Cremation in recent decades has become a popular option in place of conventional burial. Jessica Mitford in the new edition of *The American Way of Death* contends that from the time when her book was first published in 1963 until its revised edition in the late 1990s, cremation went from 3.75 percent of burial choices to 21 percent. This jump was helped along when the Catholic Church lifted its ban on cremation in the 1960s, but Mitford herself had an important role to play in changing perceptions. People who read Mitford's exposé in detail learned how funeral homes overcharge and manipulate the vulnerable; this led many to choose what they regarded as a more convenient, cheaper way to go. In Mitford's words:

> Cremation is, no doubt, a simple, tidy solution to the disposal of the
> dead. It appeals to the nature lover and the poet, who visualize their

mortal remains scattered over sunny hillside or remote strand. It is commended by environmentalists and by those who would like to see an end to all the malarkey that surrounds the usual kind of funeral.[9]

When Mitford herself died in 1996, her funeral cost $533.31. She was cremated and her ashes scattered at sea. I keep wondering about that 31 cents. But her cost-effective and environmental end has now also become almost as expensive an end-of-life option. The burning, the urn, and the scattering fees all add up. There are rental caskets to display the deceased before cremation and also costs associated with using the viewing room of the funeral home.

In the Hindu tradition of cremation, the dead body is placed on an open-air platform called a *ghat*. Lord Agni, the Hindu god of fire, is said to purify the soul. And fire, one of the five elements Hindus ascribe to a human being, is used to help detach the soul from the body because the body is reduced through burning. The fire is lit by the oldest or youngest son, depending on whether the deceased is the father or the mother, with fire from the home hearth. The child then uses a sharp instrument to break the skull to release the soul.

Cremation as we know it today in the West started in England in the nineteenth century among British intelligentsia. It was touted by the likes of George Bernard Shaw to avoid cemetery overcrowding and what he regarded as the aesthetically distasteful practice of burying people in the ground. (Of course, many East Asian religious traditions like Hinduism and Jainism have practiced cremation for thousands of years.)

Having said that, most people don't know what actually happens to the body when it is cremated, meaning the process rather than the outcome. Cremation involves burning the deceased at extremely high temperatures (roughly 700°F) until the remains—or cremains, as they are called—are reduced to ashes and bone fragments. The dead body is first deposited in a cardboard casket or container and then placed in a retort, as it is referred to in the business. The process usually takes several hours, depending on the body mass of the deceased. Legally only one body is allowed to be cremated per retort at a time. The burning is usually done in special facilities called crematoria, housed in funeral homes designed for the purpose. Some ancient traditions practice open-air burnings that are in view of family and relatives, and some conventional funeral homes allow viewing of the process as well.

Bodies react differently to the heat. Some raise their arms as the body contracts. Fat burns in different ways. Tom Jokinen, who wrote *Curtains*, worked as an undertaker-in-training and describes watching the process and later sweeping out the retort along with using the vacuum hose that sucks up human ash.

> The big and fat call for vigilance, some measure of babying and fiddling with the airflow and gas, while the small and reedy . . . are more independent and can be left alone without fear they'll burn out of control. What they ate and stored around the waistline, how fit they were, whether they had strong long-bones, the femurs and humeri, from a lifetime of manual labor—it's all relevant to the cremationist.[10]

Any metal parts, screws, staples, bridgework or false teeth do not burn and are left with the cremains. These are sorted out to leave the cleanest, whitest ash—a funeral home desirable. Human life has been reduced to basically 200 cubic inches.

Many people believe that cremation is the most sound ecological and financial method of burial. There's no property tax or shoveling fees. Even advocates of eco-burials like cremation a whole lot better than conventional burial, but they still believe that the process is too industrial and burns fossil fuels that release air pollutants. The school of more natural, organic burials does, however, like the Eternal Reef (eternalreefs.com) option, in which you take cremated ashes and mix them with concrete to shape an artificial reef form that gets added to a living coral reef and creates a new marine habitat. For about five thousand dollars, I could remain forever with my loved ones as part of a Chinese restaurant's fish tank.

I also learned about cremation diamonds as a creative way to make sure your mother is always with you, if you don't feel guilty enough already. Companies like LifeGem make memorial diamonds by taking the carbon of the cremated ashes or a piece of the deceased's hair and making a gemstone out of it for you to wear as jewelry. When they say a diamond is forever, they're not kidding. And the ads for "death jewelry" are sure to tug a few heartstrings. LifeGem has a full line of settings for cremation diamonds.

> Love. Life's single greatest risk. Life's single greatest reward. Love captures your heart in a second and holds it for eternity. You have experienced a love without equal.
>
> You have had someone truly special in your life and mere words simply will not do.

A cheaper but no less scenic option is having your ashes scattered in one of America's national parks. Permission is at the discretion of the chief ranger for each park. Permit fees range from free to $50, which does not include park entrance fees. Commercial funeral services are not allowed to scatter ashes in national parks or forests. This service is limited to private individuals. You can also pay for a hike-in service if you want your relative to be scattered somewhere more obscure in the park, but the cost multiplies, and the trips are done by rangers alone, without accompanying mourners. The company High Sierra Gardens distributes ashes in California's Sierra Nevada range for only a few hundred dollars. It can be twice that to have your ashes scattered at sea for an unaccompanied trip. Add a few hundred more dollars for a group rate if you want to go. If you're looking for something a little more tropical and exotic, try *Hawaii Ash Scatterings*, which will disperse ashes in remote areas of Oahu for less than five hundred dollars. If you never made it to Hawaii during your lifetime, there may still be a way to get there (this trip will be a lot cheaper than an airplane seat and hotel).

Many conventional cemeteries and churches now have scattering gardens or walls with plaques and markers. Cremation may have become more popular, but mourners still want to "visit" the dead; this may be an acceptable compromise.

Scattering ashes seems to obviate another niggling difficulty of traditional burials. Instead of reducing all of human life to a small plot, scattering ashes captures both the expanse and the impermanence of life. But there is a competing emotion for many when they contemplate the end: the need for containment.

In the very first chapters of the Bible, Adam is told, "By the sweat of your brow you will eat your food until you return to the ground, since from it you were taken; for dust you are and to dust you will return."[11] Even the Hebrew name "Adam" means "earth." Primordial man was a product of the earth and returned to his origins, creating a sense of finality by bookending life with the earth itself. This sentiment, often used as a cliché of funeral lingo, is taken straight from the book of Job: "Naked I came from my mother's womb, and naked I will depart."[12] Human life gets recycled, preparing the way for the next generation by "seeding" the ground that birthed the human being. Yet another famous biblical reference to the process comes from the pages of Ecclesiastes: "One generation passes away and another generation comes, but the earth abides forever. . . . All the rivers run into the sea, yet the sea is not full. Unto the place from where the rivers come, they return again."[13] The natural world, although continually in flux, endures. Human life is birthed into such a world and then collapses back into it, allowing new life to regenerate in its place. Job later makes an important distinction between the permanence of nature and the desire to be part of it and the limited, temporal life of the human being: "There is hope for a tree; if it is cut down it will renew itself; its shoots will not cease. If its roots are old in the earth, and its stump dies in the ground, at the scent of water it will bud and produce branches like a sapling. But mortals languish and die. Man expires; where is he?"[14]

We don't exactly replant the dead in cemeteries in much of the Western world today, particularly in the United States. Many of the country's largest, most well-known cemeteries were built around the same period of time, the early nineteenth century. Fearing the spread of disease created by the stacking of bodies in many churches, especially during medical epidemics, independent burial societies developed the notion of large cemeteries on the outskirts of town. The idea was to give the dead "space." What it really offered was some psychic freedom and bacterial relief from the poor hygienic conditions of the eighteenth century. It was the living who really wanted the space apart from the dead.

This is a far cry from some of the celebrity cemeteries of today, the most famous of which is probably Forest Lawn in Hollywood Hills. Beautiful people should keep the right company even when they are no longer able to have company. And yes, just as there are maps of Hollywood that tell you where the stars live, there are maps available of Forest Lawn to tell you where *their* celebrities live; famous names like Lucille Ball, Gene Autry, Bette Davis and, my favorite, Liberace, reside in Forest Lawn. I could only imagine what Liberace might have wanted for his resting place. But why imagine when you can actually visit? Liberace died in 1987 of AIDS (although he denied it with his last breath and fought court battles to deny his homosexuality). He is memorialized in the park in the Court of Remembrance with a large crypt where he, his mother and his brother George are interred. On top of the white marble crypt is a classic Greek statue of a woman, and on the front carved into the marble is an image of his famous piano and candelabra and Liberace's signature. It was attention-grabbing but certainly less garish than I expected. I guess that was saved for the now shuttered Liberace Museum in Las Vegas.

If we could design our own eternal resting place with no expense spared, would we go the Liberace route? I don't think I would. I tend to dress in a more understated way, but I do understand the temptation. The writer Hans Morgenthau observes that the need to memorialize a life is a powerful manifestation of the human condition: "Man on all levels of civilization is moved to create monuments which testify to his existence and will live after him. . . . Over his grave he causes a monument of stone to be erected whose durability, as it were, compensates for the importance of what lies beneath."[15] We need to capture our own uniqueness. We have to mark that place, sometimes forever or with the belief that our mark will last forever. This is the call to immortality that is often an aphrodisiac for the creative and the gifted. The perpetual escape clause from death lies in the possibility that something you do or write or paint will outlive you and therefore you will live on through it, avoiding death of a metaphysical kind, avoiding extinction. And if not, there is always the two-tier marble crypt.

With all of the destination locations we might pick for a final vacation, I wondered why we most often stick with boring cemeteries. In the years since Alyssa's burial, I have spoken with people who had anxieties about conventional burials in cemeteries, but most people never really entertain the notion of being put anywhere else when the time comes. We're not too creative about death. It seems that a cemetery is the most natural, most anticipated space option for the dead. Most cemeteries even seem peaceful and inviting, enveloping us in their silence without the Styrofoam Halloween RIP-tombstone-look that is stereotypically associated with gravesites.

But as we think about it, it does seem rather odd the way that the dead have their own neighborhoods, usually living separately from the living on the periphery of our towns, in long expanses of neatly manicured grave estates that offer the dead room that they hardly need. After all, dying isn't like football; you don't actually need a big field.

Cemeteries are probably one of the most remarkable, sanctified spaces in any town, place of worship or military enclave. Tombstones are like bookmarks on the verdant field of history. Meandering through them takes you back in time: died young, died after a long life, died only a few months after his wife. We begin to write stories in our minds about people, stories that we can rarely verify.

In days gone by, people buried family members right on the family property. Your dearest stayed nearest. But why bury at all? Burying the dead in the ground probably dates back to Neanderthal man, between 20,000 and 75,000 years ago. Hunters used to bury the dead in the ground or in caves to protect the bodies from wild animals, generally on an east-west axis, with the head facing east. This ritual is still practiced by the Greek Orthodox today. As rituals around the dead developed in agrarian societies, people may have been buried in the ground as a way of "re-planting" them in the hopes of symbolically re-populating the world or bringing the dead back through the life-cycle of vegetation.

What many want, a return to nature, is not unlike a new trend in cemeteries (which seems an awful lot like an old trend). It's called eco-burial. Eco-burial grounds are also known as woodland cemeteries, green cemeteries, memorial nature preserves or natural burial grounds. The idea is to use only biodegradable materials in the burial of a person: no chemical preservatives are used in the preparation of the body, just simple wooden caskets, recyclable paper caskets (often covered in notes from loved ones), or no caskets at all and only degradable shrouds. Usually a tree or a shrub is planted over the actual grave to mark the place rather than a headstone. Sometimes flat markers contain information on the dead so that nothing intrudes on the patterns of nature. Sometimes no markers are used. When I learned that, I thought of Anton Chekhov, who once considered why people write graffiti in natural settings:

> When a man in a melancholy mood is left tête-à-tête with the sea, or any landscape which seems to him grandiose, there is always, for some reason, mixed with melancholy, a conviction that he will live and die in obscurity, and he reflectively snatches up a pencil and hastens to write his name on the first thing that comes handy.[16]

Humans need to mark nature precisely because we feel so small in relation to it. Concerns that the body will "disappear" in an eco-burial ground because it is not overtly marked are allayed by the use of a modern survey technique called GIS (geographic information system) to locate the place of each interment with precision. Chekhov triumphs.

The Centre for Natural Burial says that natural burial began in 1993. I don't know how they arrived at that date. I thought it started twenty millennia ago, at least. But they make a compelling case when they question what today's conventional burial techniques and methods do to our planet:

> With a typical modern funeral, the body is laid naked on a stainless steel embalmer's table, bled out, and pumped full of noxious

chemicals to keep the body fresh. Following the viewing, the body is sealed inside a metal casket or lacquered wooden coffin lined with plush satin and adorned with beautiful brass accessories . . . which is then lowered into a concrete vault and buried.

The reinforced concrete tomb is covered with a ton of dirt, and planted with a monoculture of grass which is kept artificially green with pest and weed killer. Above ground, the local cemetery may look pastoral and natural; however, below the surface it serves to all intents and purposes as a landfill of hazardous wastes and non-biodegradable materials.[17]

The Centre claims that when it comes to most conventional burials, the process takes more than a week and will cost heirs a small fortune. Green burial costs are generally between $1,000 and $4,000 depending on the cost of transporting the body and if there is an engraved marker of some kind. The fees include a plot of land, the cost of opening and closing the grave, a stone marker and sustainability costs to make sure that the area is properly tended. This bargain-basement cost does not include any memorial service fees. It's just the basics. At first I thought that was cheap, but then I wondered why it costs anything at all if you want to be buried, let's say, in your own backyard. Your family could visit all of the time, and you would still have the comforts of home, in a really weird sense. It seems like a perfectly good solution to at least one fear of the unknown: will I spend my eternal life surrounded by strangers? One Alabama resident, Jim Davis, decided that he loved his wife, Patsy, so much he was going to bury her in the front lawn. Why hide her in the back?[18] He checked and there was no local ordinance against it in the city of Stevenson, where he lives. There have been some complaints about property values and the protracted controversy is not over, but so far, it is not illegal.

• • •

All of the burial options confused me. I must confess that it's hard to read about cremation when members of my family were gassed and put in ovens at concentration camps throughout Eastern Europe. I acknowledge my bias. Still, as I learned about cremation and all of the funky ways I could be disposed of, it became harder to get Fadwa and Cheryl out of my mind and the way they revere the human body, the way their faith commitments acknowledge the presence of death as a sacred reality. No one is trying to put death off or hide it away. There is no violence done to the body for the sake of a "memory picture" for the living. The often brutal treatment the body sustains from a trocar, in a retort or through chemical injection seems to go against the very fiber of what most people are trying to create in death: a serene and tranquil send-off. I think of a line in *Curtains* when the author, having spent months as an undertaker-in-training who learned how to use a retort and a trocar, turns to his wife and says, "I have seen the future . . . and it's Jewish."[19]

The funeral-home industry presents a clean, sanitized version of death rather than acknowledging it as the mess that it is. I keep returning to the love, grace and compassion of volunteers like Fadwa and Cheryl, who remind me of Ralph Waldo Emerson's words: "Peace cannot be achieved through violence; it can only be attained through understanding." In Islam and Judaism and other faiths that encounter death straight on, there are no injections, no elaborate makeup or fancy dressing up of the dead. There is the body, a simple yet holy vessel that returns to the ground and lets the soul fly free. When I go, whenever that is, I want to know and want my family to know that someone will lovingly care for my body as it leaves this world and becomes part of the ground. From dust to dust.

• • •

The walk through the cemetery that hot morning when Diane, Roy and I were looking for plots prompted me to wonder about the connection between burial spaces and happier endings. Does knowing where you will be buried make it easier to overcome your fear of death? Yes, it seems to. Having some visual location in mind eases the fright of death as a black hole. "This is where I will live one day" does offer a modicum of solace and is another reason to purchase plots well in advance of their use. Knowing how your body will be treated and where it will go offers a glimpse of control in an otherwise uncontrollable set of circumstances.

This part of my quest for the better end helped me work through some intense fears about what will happen to my body after I go. I know I will not be around to judge the experience either way, but my survivors should feel reassured that, just as I came into this world already loved, I exit it embraced with sanctity and love. I am reminded of a teaching of the Talmudic sage Rabbi Meir. He once said, "When you come into the world your hands are clenched, as if to say: the whole world is mine and I will inherit it. And when you take leave of the world your hands are open, as if to say: I have not taken from this world a single thing."[20] Sure, there is something liberating about the thought of my ashes being scattered in a beautiful place. But I want the security of containment. After spending a lifetime grabbing for things and experiences to mark the fact that I was here, I want to surrender myself to death, to the groundedness of the earth. That is what I leave for my survivors: a place where the remains, and then only the marker, will reside. I think of what C. S. Lewis once said: "You don't have a soul. You are a soul. You have a body." And when I depart this world, I will thank my body for housing my soul and treating it with the utmost dignity as it goes back to the place whence it came. I offer my gratitude.

## Chapter Four

# Death as an Escape

One of the great unanswered questions about my cousin Alyssa's death was why it ever happened. She was not medically ill, nor were there overt signs of depression. She left no note. Of course, the police had to ask if she was suicidal, and, as a family, the issue came up. But the guess was most likely that, no, she did not take her own life. The enigma of it all was deeply unsettling. It got in the way of any closure.

We all know that death is an escape for those who willfully choose it. Alyssa may not have made that choice, but it is not an irrational one. In my quest to understand happier endings, I had to come to terms with suicide. It seemed to be a happier ending for those who selected it and a very unhappy ending for the survivors. Who gets to choose?

Suicide for many is a rational decision, not an impulsive act of darkness. In perhaps the most "rational" depiction of suicide, Christopher Buckley's 2007 novel *Boomsday* offered a sci-fi future world where senior citizens can opt for suicide for financial incentives when turning seventy in order to spare their children and society from having to support them. Additional bonuses were available for those willing to die at sixty-five. Buckley calls this "voluntary transitioning." It is an amusing concept until it isn't, and the full fright of a brave new world on a slippery slope appears before us. It is not as giant a leap from the rational decision to end a life to *Boomsday* as we might have imagined.

If my quest was to have any authenticity, I had to ask a strange question: is taking one's life a way to overcome the fear of death? It seems that for the restless and unhappy, suicide is the only truly happy ending; it prevents one from having to face the pain of another day. This became abundantly clear to me some years ago on a day that still rattles me.

I was at work. It was a typical day of meetings and e-mail correspondence when I heard the gallop of shoes and saw, in my peripheral vision, one of the managing directors of our office race down the corridor of our fourth floor. Why was she running? I peeked my head out into the hallway to see what was going on and saw the senior leadership team quickly slide into a room and then slam a door shut. Something was happening that the rest of us were not privy to—yet.

One of the rising stars in our organization had taken his life at age twenty-six. Marc uncharacteristically failed to show up at a meeting and did not respond to calls on his cell or house phone. Finally, understanding that perhaps something was gravely wrong, a few coworkers went to his apartment. He was dead. No explanation. No note. No forewarning.

By the time the news broke in the office, I was already picking up my children from school. There was an emergency staff meeting to let everyone know. Grief counselors were at hand. The CEO called me at home. Marc was a friend. The CEO knew we were close. I hung up the phone and went outside to sit on my porch step, crying and trying to grasp how a beautiful young soul had died alone in an apartment. There are so many things that I will never understand, and at that moment I had one more item on my list of universal and painful mysteries.

I walked inside, sat down, and held my three-year-old on my lap, feeling with amazing clarity what it means to hold on tightly to the ones we love. She asked me why my face looked funny, and I told her I was sad. She asked me if I was sad at her, and I said no.

"But why are you sad?" she persisted.

"I had a friend named Marc. I am not going to see him anymore, and I miss him already."

Marc was Swiss by birth, and he decided to remain in America after graduating from college. Our organization sponsored his citizenship. Marc had a big smile and a funny, awkward laugh; combined with his lanky figure, bushy eyebrows and dark-rimmed glasses, he had that cool nerd look. Many older colleagues described him as another son, the one they wished they had. He was the first person to take me out to lunch, a lovely practice he had with all new colleagues. One married woman in our office wrote in his memorial book that when he asked her to lunch, just to be friendly, she mistook it for a date. She later felt embarrassed because it was just Marc's way of being nice. Even at his young age, Marc understood how to welcome people and make them feel at home, even in a place that was not his native home. One of our staff nailed it when she said, "Marc is my favorite type of person. Too smart for his own good, stubborn as hell and damn good at debating. Yes, with Marc, while he may not have been right, he was never wrong. And yet his awkward hunched gait, hands in pockets, smile hidden, made me want to give him a hug so hard, he'd lose his breath."

If Marc was struggling with mental illness or living with a dark cloud over him, I never saw it. The news of his suicide was dizzying. There must have been a mistake.

I went down one floor to Marc's office the next day. His papers were a mess. He was in the middle of several projects. He hadn't cleaned his desk. This somehow had a vast impact on my incapacity to process his death. It's the same warped thinking that produced the motherly advice to wear clean underwear just in case something happens to you. Clad in a pair of clean underwear, there will be nothing bad someone can say about you if you die. Surprisingly, I have never heard anyone eulogize a dead person with the memorable words: "At least he was wearing clean underwear when they found him after the accident." In the same perverse line of thinking, when I go on vacation, my house has to be spotless so that if anything happens to me while I'm gone, whoever enters my house for my personal effects will know that I was an orderly person. In my limited mind, I could only imagine a person leaving this world with a clean desk.

And there was one small detail that I cannot erase from that visit. When I stroked the rounded corners of Marc's desk, as if to ask this inanimate object to explain what really happened, I noticed that he had a tall paper cup from a convenience store on the desk; it had a straw in it. Marc could not possibly be dead because some of his now flat soda was still there, with a straw, for goodness' sake.

A few weeks later, I spoke at Marc's memorial service. His parents came from Switzerland, traversing an abyss of grief to be with us and remember their son. I did not look at anyone when I took the podium. A career of studying and teaching religious texts had not prepared me for the moment ahead. I spoke of Marc's wry sense of humor, his seriousness of purpose, his reliability and his deep sense of mission. I told his parents that it would be impossible to detail all of the people he touched and the ways that he served others, an enviable list of accomplishments people far older than Marc had yet to achieve. When I finished, Marc's father got up to thank everyone for being Marc's family and community and for mourning him that way. As I passed his dad on the way down, I collapsed into his arms, the arms of a stranger. I felt the ground under my feet shake. I lost my composure.

Marc's office has had many other occupants over the years, but it will always be his in my mind. The mess of papers, the cup, the straw. I cannot walk into that room without feeling that this never should have happened and should never happen again.

Marc's death was another turning point for me as a person and an educator. It seemed, suddenly, as if every spiritual text and tradition, every ritual pointed ultimately to death in some way. Life will be meaningful only if death stands before us as a stop sign, forcing us to confront life's most difficult conversations, enabling us to dig deeper into the well of wisdom and empowering us to search for transcendence in the everyday business of living. Marc put unhappy endings into hyperfocus for me. Their suddenness. The lack of explanation. The conundrum. The heartache. The missing note. The question mark that was Marc's absence. Many years later, I asked our chief of staff if she had more information. I aimed for a closure that was destined to elude me. "We just don't know." Knowledge doesn't change death. It doesn't make it more acceptable. I don't know what I was after. Was there any piece of information that would have changed the loss? I doubt it.

Marc was not my first personal encounter with suicide, just the one that felt closest, the one that made me pay attention to suicide differently, the one that made me wonder, when I meet someone who seems happy and friendly, what demons lurk within that I cannot see, and made me question how powerful those demons are. Formerly suspect of curmudgeons, I was suddenly wary of those who seemed too cheery. I wanted to know what was hidden beneath. I paid fresh attention to stories in the news involving suicide. And one turned up that, like Marc's, made me wonder what it would have been like to be a parent or a girlfriend in this narrative of otherness.

A Sudanese girl is squatting on the ground, her body ravaged by starvation, her arms splayed out from her sides like the wings of a bird. I am haunted by this photograph, which I saw in the Newseum in Washington, D.C. It was part of an exhibit that probed the ethics of journalism. In the foreground of the photo, the girl's posture is mimicked ominously by a vulture that awaits her last breath; its wings too are spread out. The photojournalist, Kevin Carter, who was born in South Africa during apartheid, had waited twenty minutes for the alignment of child and bird. It was one of the world's first exposures to the dangers of life in the Sudan, and for this photo, Carter won the Pulitzer Prize. Hundreds of people contacted the *New York Times* to find out the fate of the young girl. A Florida newspaper saw it a little bit differently: "The man adjusting his lens to take just the right frame of her suffering, might just as well be a predator, another vulture on the scene."

Carter returned to the United States and wrestled with the human cost of his award-winning photo and the battle with death he constantly photographed. Twenty minutes of his assistance, instead of twenty minutes waiting for the shot, may have saved this child. He could not live with himself; a few years later, Carter took his own life. In some way, Carter had responded to Albert Camus's famous statement in *The Myth of Sisyphus*: "There is but one truly serious philosophical problem, and that is suicide. Judging whether life is or is not worth living amounts to answering the fundamental question of philosophy."[1] Carter answered the fundamental question of philosophy in the only way he could. Life for him was not worth living, and he was to be the judge of himself.

Suicide is a profound decision. For those who struggle with daily existence and the nightmare of unhappy future prospects, living another day in a world that hurts is a difficult choice. The American comedian Bill Maher has an interesting approach to people battling this dilemma: "Suicide is our way of saying to God, 'You can't fire me. I quit.'" In Maher's words, suicide sounds empowering. It is our only real way of controlling what happens to us when we decide that life as we know it is just not worth it. The ancient Stoic philosopher Seneca would have agreed: "The wise man will live as long as he ought, not as long as he can. . . . [He] always reflects concerning the quality, not the quantity, of his life. As soon as there are many events in his life that give him trouble and disturb his peace of mind, he sets himself free."[2] Carter set himself free, unburdening himself of all the pain, much like a person who opens a window and allows a bird to fly far away.

Try Seneca's reasoning on the wife of a man who committed suicide one afternoon while she was at work, or speak to the parents of a teenager who wrestled with his self-worth and jumped off a bridge. None would be coddled by the thought that the end ended his or her suffering. They might not be consoled by the glib quotes of modern or ancient philosophers.

But can't this be considered a happy ending if it was expressly wanted by the sufferer? He stopped fighting his failures; his suffering is finally over. She found rest; a burden lifted from her family. The outcome of ending suffering is not happy per se, but it is happier than prolonged misery.

In *What Dying People Want*, David Kuhl writes that physician-assisted suicide (which is illegal in Canada and the United States, except in Oregon) is often regarded as a relief for those facing terminal illness. The fear of unknown pain in the future can make a dying person reconsider notions of autonomy in the present. "Most people don't want to die, but some explore to varying degrees what it might mean to end their suffering by committing suicide."[3] Kuhl shares the difficult professional moment of visiting a twenty-six-year-old patient with testicular cancer who had been fighting chronic pain for years. The months and months of agony became overwhelming; one day he was rushed to the hospital because of excruciating pain. Kuhl arrived at his bedside, and the young man grabbed his doctor's arm and implored, "David, please just kill me, kill me! I can't take it anymore."[4]

It is impossible not to have compassion at such a moment and believe that what a dying person says should be taken at face value, as a request to stop forcing life when life doesn't work the way that we want it to. Kuhl recognizes, however, that the request to end life is not the same as the request to end pain, and that the two are often confused. For most people, pain relief can be achieved at a much less dramatic cost.

End-of-life wishes highlight the difference between pain and suffering. Pain is an immediate sensation that indicates that all is not well in terms of our physical health. A persistent ache in a tooth cries out for attention; a kidney stone rages within us until it passes; an ear pulses with stabbing vibrations when it is infected. The philosopher Ludwig Wittgenstein believed that pain is one of the most solitary of human experiences. It not only hurts us. It isolates us from others. When a friend says, "Oh, I also have a toothache," we don't believe for a moment that it is as severe as our own. The intensity of physical pain can have an ambush affect; pain totally takes over our human ecosystem, making it virtually impossible to think about anything else: to do our work, to focus on our children's needs, to read a book.

Responsibilities and pleasures are hijacked by physical torments, and under pain's influence it is hard to believe that the discomfort will ever go away. The negativity, intensity and totality of physical or mental misery, particularly when it is of unknown duration, can drive people to speed up the trajectory of death.

Most religious and Western traditions, however, do not regard suicide as a positive ending or a reasoned choice. Living in a society strongly influenced by Judeo-Christian ethics, we are culturally conditioned to reject suicide. Within a religious framework, suicide is an affront and insult to God's creation. If we are all made in God's image, then suicide robs God and the world of what is a divinely created and inspired being. The person who takes her life, in this spiritual scheme, has essentially failed to find the divine spark within her or is rejecting God's purpose for her as well as rejecting the self.

But this tidy summation is not true to the complexity of suicide and what motivates it, even among adherents to religious traditions that promote such a view. Every day people disregard these obstacles in the quest for nonselfhood.

Anna Karenina is perhaps the most famous literary escape into death. Anna, involved in petty jealousies, addicted to morphine and trying to get back at her lover, Vronsky, decides to leave her worries by putting an end to it all. "Yes, I'm very much worried, and that's what reason was given me for, to escape; so then one must escape: why not put out the light when there's nothing more to look at, when it's sickening to look at it at all? But how?"

Her question is not the existentialist "why" but the pragmatic "how." Reason, not emotion, dictates her thinking, and reason tells her to put an end to it all. Having first met Vronsky at a train station when a worker was killed on the tracks, Anna stands at the tracks contemplating her own death as an escape from a life riddled with self-induced suffering. We stand at the edge of the platform with her, wondering what she will decide. Suddenly, Tolstoy tells us, "she knew what to do."

But alas, as with so many suicide attempts, her timing is off, and she misses the moment; she tries to fling herself under the wheels of the first train carriage but is delayed by her red bag. She fails to drop it fast enough. We can almost see the bag, the small, vivid detail getting in the way of this momentous decision. Anna crosses herself and, with that small gesture from her past, "life rose up before her for an instant with all its bright joys." We sense a reprieve on the emotional horizon. But Tolstoy forbids us this comfort. Anna falls on her knees on the track, asks, "Where am I? What am I doing? What for?" as something "huge and merciless struck her on the head." She says, "Lord forgive me all," and then whatever light she saw went out.

Anna's escape would not be called by most a happy ending. And yet, she conceives of it as a natural end to suffering, and in that respect, suicide becomes an act of autonomy and control. Relatives and friends of a person who committed suicide often believe that the end was somehow anticipated or even a relief that stopped the everyday anguish of facing another day: "He finally found peace." The emotional torment has ceased. In actuality, he did not find peace (or may have—we will never know). He created a state of oblivion that prevented the constant or near-constant psychic battle he faced from recurring. And his peace may have come at the price of emotional unrest for those who are left forevermore with heartache and unanswered questions.

Today Anna would not have to resort to the violence of a train death. She could have checked into Dignitas, a clinic and support group in Switzerland that provides services for those who are terminally ill or just weary of life and want to end it all on their own terms, almost. Dignitas offers one way to go. After you've signed all your papers and spent a few days in the clinic, you can elect to go into a small room and take two vials. The first is filled with a serum to prevent you from throwing up the second vial. The second vial is filled with a poison. You will most likely fall asleep from the pentobarbital within ten minutes. Respiratory arrest usually follows within a half-hour. There is a camera in the room making sure that the helper who is there to assist you is not forcing your hand in any way. If this is an autonomous decision, then every part of it must be self-determined, down to the opening of the poison vial that will put an end to it all.

We have made much of Jack Kevorkian in the United States, but Dignitas has moved the whole project of assisted suicide out of the covert, illegal and shadowy reputation of Kevorkian-like procedures to a proper choice. It was founded by Ludwig Minelli in 1998, and it does not provide death services like a fast-food drive-through. Independent doctors make assessments of the mental stability of those coming to Dignitas. All clients must be, according to a licensed psychiatrist, *compos mentis* and have a signed affidavit; if they are no longer able to sign a document of informed consent, they can make a video with the same intent. The cost of the service ranges depending on whether or not the client opts for additional funeral services, but the price tag is roughly between $5,000 and $12,000 (U.S.). If you are coming from another country—what is affectionately dubbed suicide tourism (from John Zaritsky's documentary *The Suicide Tourist*)—add on the rental fees of Dignitas apartments while all the paperwork is prepared and the medical exams are conducted.

The English writer Terry Pratchett is trying to get a similar facility built in England. Pratchett has early onset Alzheimer's disease, and he made a documentary in 2011 called *Terry Pratchett: Choosing to Die*, in which he takes his audience through an assisted suicide at Dignitas. With permission, he followed an Englishman through the process, and, in true English fashion, the man thanked everyone there for coming before he ingested his poison. In an NPR interview, Pratchett basically called assisted suicide a happy ending: "I believe that everyone should have a good death. You know, with your grandchildren around you, a bit of sobbing. Because, after all, tears are appropriate on a deathbed. And you say goodbye to your loved ones, making certain that one of them has been left behind to look after the shop."[5]

Pratchett, in his global campaign to make death choices more autonomous, believes we should move away from the word "suicide" because it smacks too much of irrationalism. The people he has met who have favored this option are all very rational people, he claims. So are their families. People facing terminal illness believe it is an absolutely reasonable decision to end it all rather than "spend any more time than necessary in the jaws of the beast." Although Pratchett believes in assisted suicide for the terminally ill, he is less supportive of those who come to Dignitas because they are simply tired of living. Everyone has those moments, he believes, and if he had acted on them, there would be books he wouldn't have written and loves he wouldn't have had. After all, how much are we like our "real" selves at darker times when the world seems bleak and unbearable? This more swampy issue complicates everything. According to statistics about Dignitas clients, just over 20 percent fall into the "weary of life" category. They are not terminally ill, just terminally sick of living. Dignitas has not been very transparent about costs and clientele, and, although it is a nonprofit, it does not publicize a good deal of information about its inner workings. Consequently, it has come under fire, most recently from an ex-employee who has shared a bit of the shadier side of the business of death at Dignitas, claiming financial irregularities and a lack of transparency when there are problems with the procedure.

Pratchett's campaign focuses on the terminally ill and the lack of choices they have. His support of assisted suicide may very well come from personal experience. He was contacted too late to witness the death of his mother, and he was disturbed by the long, drawn-out death of his father. He did not feel it was a bad death, just a prolonged encounter with morphine. "Frankly they could have been more frank with us, and frank with him. And what was the point? It wore my mother out, I think."[6]

As for himself, Pratchett worries that with Alzheimer's he may not be in full mental health to make the decision when it's time. But it's not time yet. As Pratchett says, "I'm a writer who's writing books, and therefore I don't want to die. You'd miss the end of the book, wouldn't you? . . . You can't die with an unfinished book."[7]


That is not true, strictly speaking: you can die with an unfinished book. There are plenty of authors who die midnovel or with a work of nonfiction not completed. Yet the journalist and *New York* magazine critic Sam Anderson claims that the human brain automatically finishes unfinished things, like joining together the ends of an incomplete circle or filling in the missing letter of a word. We have a deep psychological need to complete that which is incomplete. Anderson claims that we do the same with unfinished novels. We can't bear the thought that an author would leave this world with pages unwritten. Rationally, why should we give authors a different, more privileged sort of end than we give, say, accountants who die in mid-tax season and, therefore, did not have the time to fill out every form for every client? Yet Anderson claims that we just can't stand to know that an author has died midwork. When it comes to a novel,

> we always end up finishing them with *something*. We fill in the blanks, unconsciously, with what is closest at hand: the gestalt, the legend, the vibe, the tone, the aesthetic of the author in question.

This is, after all, what a great author does: he trains us not just to receive his vision but also to extend it—to read the world (its landscapes, people, events, texts) in the peculiar way that he would have read them. He *infuses* the world, almost like a religion (after a few Dickens novels, everything starts to look Dickensian). So it makes sense that we would carry that vision to an author's own last work.[8]

Anderson claims that most authors who die were probably still intending to write something, but "mortality and ambition rarely coincide." This is particularly painful when the author has the desire to complete a novel or even to begin one but his mind is failing or her body is just not functional enough to offer the physical strength necessary. The author David Foster Wallace, for example, committed suicide but left, on his desk, twelve completed chapters of a novel neatly stacked with the remaining hundreds of pages in various stages of completion and revision in notes and files. The organized pile of work was read as an invitation to collate the rest of the writerly mess into the manuscript of the book now called *The Pale King*, which was released in 2011, two and a half years after the author died. We can easily imagine someone reading such a book, even if a true Wallace fan may feel despair at something she feels (but will never know) was done by a Wallace impostor determined to finish that which was intentionally left unfinished. Wallace knew exactly what he left for others, something undercooked.

It's hard to imagine reviewing such a book—although it has been reviewed. An unfinished book feels like the parroting of an unfinished life or even the tease that the author puts out for his reading public so that people will truly miss him when he's gone. There may be no way to finish a life and take care of every little detail.

But Dudley Clendinen tried to do just that. Clendinen, a former national correspondent and editorial writer for the *New York Times,* described his intentional choice to end his life when he learned he had amyotrophic lateral sclerosis (ALS), otherwise known as Lou Gehrig's disease, after the Yankee hitter who died from the disease at age thirty-eight. Clendinen stopped calling it "Gehrig's disease" in favor of "Lou," since it felt more familiar and less threatening to call a fatal illness by its first name. When Clendinen let his friends know he was dying, one friend flew in from Texas and quietly said, "We need to go buy you a pistol, don't we?" Instead of getting upset, Clendinen agreed.

Clendinen had spent hundreds of hours at his mother's side when she was dying, and she barely recognized him. He did not want that future for his own daughter. So he decided to end his life when he determined the time was right. He respected people who choose to suffer until the end, but it wasn't a choice he felt comfortable with. He tabulated the expense, the quality of life, the challenges the late stages of Lou would have for him and his family, and it just didn't add up. He felt that we talk about everything, "but we don't talk about how to die. We act as if facing death weren't one of life's greatest, most absorbing thrills and challenges. . . . It is. This is not dull."[9]

Understanding what will happen to him medically prompted Clendinen to make his decision:

> I'd rather die. I respect the wishes of people who want to live as long as they can. But I would like the same respect for those of us who de-cide—rationally—not to. I've done my homework. I have a plan. . . . I just have to act while my hands still work: the gun, narcotics, sharp blades, a plastic bag, a fast car, over-the-counter drugs, oleander tea (the polite Southern way), carbon monoxide, even helium. That would give me a *really* funny voice at the end.[10]

He did not make these observations with anger but with a voice of reason, even humor. There may have been fear behind that voice that we couldn't hear, but Clendinen wanted to take the sting out of death and the conventional belief that death will come when it wills, not when we will it. *New York Times* columnist David Brooks was clearly moved by Clendinen's piece and tied it into our failing health care system:

> Years ago, people hoped that science could delay the onset of morbidity. We would live longer, healthier lives and then die quickly. This is not happening. Most of us will still suffer from chronic diseases for years near the end of life, and then die slowly.[11]

We have created, very possibly, the worst of all possible worlds when it comes to death and aging: we have the capacity to keep people alive longer than they can maintain a desirable quality of life.

We understand Clendinen's motives and Dignitas confirms them; suicide is perhaps the greatest expression of personal autonomy. Nothing can be more intimate or more self-directed than the decision to end one's life by choice. This may be a good death in the sense that it is a controlled ending. But the pain for those left behind lies in the possibility, however remote, that whatever black cloud shadowed this person's life could have been removed and a permanent state of happiness could have been achieved. That possibility will be continually mulled over by those who remain. And can a death ever be considered good if it is only judged that way by one person?

Taking a journey back in time to answer this question, we visit the devastation of students over a teacher who had one of the most famous assisted suicides of all time: Socrates. His death has become the object of myth, legend and art precisely because Socrates used his death to teach those around him about true autonomy: the right to live for what one believes in, even if that means compromising that life by dying for one's cause. Socrates' death is described at the end of Plato's *Phaedo*. Socrates turned down the pleas of Crito, his old friend, to attempt an escape from prison. The philosopher would not listen, because escaping would violate the verdict determined by the citizens of Athens at his trial in 399 BCE. Crito visited him frequently in prison and could not believe the way in which his friend accepted death with equanimity. On one such visit, Plato tells of Crito's early-morning trip to the prison, when he waited for the famous Athenian to wake up:

> **Crito:** I did not wake you on purpose, so that you could continue so pleasantly. Both often and before in all your life you have had a happy disposition, and especially now in your present misfortune, you bear it so easily and mildly.
> **Socrates:** Surely, Crito, it would be a mistake at my age to resent it if I must die now.

When the day finally arrived for Socrates to meet his death, he drank the hemlock and was told to walk until it took effect. It numbed him and was traveling to his heart as he spoke to his devoted friend for the very last time: "Crito, we owe a rooster to Asclepius. Please, don't forget to pay the debt." This odd message has been interpreted in any number of ways. Asclepius was the god of illness; perhaps Socrates wanted to give the god thanks for releasing him from the burden of this lifetime where truth was not allowed to flourish. The famous last line of the *Apology* is "I go to die and you to live; who knows which is the better journey?"

When Jacques-Louis David painted *The Death of Socrates*, he shook up eighteenth-century French society. Instead of lying calmly and going to his death with his cup of poison, Socrates sits upright in the composition; the ankle chain that once fettered this free thinker to the bed is broken and snakes across the floor. Near it lies a scroll that perhaps held some of the philosopher's wisdom or may have held his indictment. The sage is bathed in light and holds his left arm upright with a finger pointing heavenward. Relief awaits.

Several disciples look reverentially at Socrates; one cups his head in his hands in grief. Two hold on to the gray stone walls as if the world itself were collapsing. Others turn their gaze away, unable to navigate the difficult emotions of the moment. In the background a few people walk up the stairs of what looks like an underground dungeon, leaving the philosopher alone to share an emotional parting with his beloved students. The figure in the composition's center wears a red tunic that mirrors the red cup of poison Socrates will soon drink. He too turns his face away and covers his eyes as he holds the hemlock out; Socrates' right hand hovers above the cup. The onlooker understands that this death is unwanted but dignified. Socrates may have been put to death but he would die animatedly, taking his death in his own hands and speaking wisdom with his very last breath. The artist himself may have had a personal agenda; he was an active supporter of the French Revolution and was imprisoned after Robespierre's fall from power. Standing up for the truth was worth it, even to the death. Death in this painting is a powerful, personal statement of defiance.

Socrates was put to death for questioning Athenian politics and society, but he died willingly and with dignity. He sought no escape route and died on principle. If what John Webster said in 1612 is true—that death has "ten thousand several doors"—dignity may just be a preferred exit in which to meet the grim reaper. Socrates wanted his disciples to understand the meaning of conviction but, at the same time, left them with an unanswered question: to die or to live—which is the better option?

• • •

Few people will die the famous death of Socrates. But many of us have heard a friend or relative say, "If I ever get that sick, just shoot me on the spot." The way the remark is phrased suggests that the burden will be placed on others. "Shoot me," they ask, as if that's a responsibility someone else would welcome in such a situation. At least Dudley Clendinen was prepared to do himself in and didn't expect his friends to do the dirty work. While we sympathize with his anguish, we also know that there is another side to the suicide equation: most of those left behind never would have wanted the deceased to make the choice. The philosopher C. G. Prado observes that while those who choose to die through suicide, assisted suicide or euthanasia may have come to terms with their decision after agonizing over it, the same may not be true of their friends and relatives.

The people who surround the dying often have to make painful psychological adjustments to match their religious or cultural sensibilities to a new reality of death by choice. This may place a heavy and unanticipated weight on them that could last a lifetime. Guilt, remorse, confusion and self-judgment often become associated with their relationship to the dead in such circumstances. The deceased becomes more than a bundle of memories, good and bad; that person becomes an open-ended question in the mind of those he or she left behind. What if she got better? What if a cure is found soon? Did he know what he was doing? Couldn't we have found a way to lessen the pain? Shouldn't I have told him . . . ? What if . . . ?

Prado questions the moral and emotional responsibility that electors (his term for those who voluntarily opt to die) have to survivors. We are human beings, after all, and despite the reasoned arguments an elector offers, we cannot sever our emotional attachments to the person we love and care for, and we are not always willing to accept irrevocable choices. Prado notes the degree of selfishness or perception of selfishness that such a choice represents to survivors; those who actively seek death because life is not viable for them often cannot see beyond their own suffering to realize that they may be an agent of suffering for those they love:

> Opting to die rather than endure terminal illness is an inherently self-interested and self-absorbed choice, and it is naïve to deny that it is. Choosing to die means serving one's own interests first, even if one does so by forgoing life itself. And choosing to die inexorably means relinquishing relationships with others, and that is something that of course is done before life is actually ended.[12]

Prado claims that it is common for those who elect to die to begin a process of distancing themselves, consciously or unconsciously, from friends and relatives because of their sharpened focus on themselves and their situation. The needs, feelings and concerns of others begin to drop from the view of the elector, particularly in the case of terminal illness, because such conditions consume so much physical and emotional energy. This actually helps the elector separate from those around him when making this ultimate choice.

The survivors, on the other hand, do not make a similar emotional journey and instead slowly detach themselves from the elector out of anger or resentment while the elector is still living, because the decision to die is also a decision to end all relationships; as such, it can become a secret poison between two otherwise loving people. It signals—even if unintentionally—a rejection of the other. "If you loved me, you would never do this to me." Festering silence or heated exchanges take the place of the tender farewells that the elector hoped for when making the choice to die: "Choosing to die to escape an anguished and hopeless existence is, after all, effectively to choose to end all relationships and one's life."[13] And this is only in the instance where the choice to die is made known to others in advance. When it is not, the emotional severance of the relationship can feel sharp and unyielding in its unspoken criticism of that relationship.

Prado suggests that electors, to be remembered lovingly by their survivors, may opt to extend life simply "for the sake of mutual affection and commitment," as a way of minimizing self-absorption and not putting an end to relationships.[14] This is a sacrifice on the part of the elector, but there will always be a sacrifice; the question is, who is to make the sacrifice?

Selfishness may manifest itself on both sides of the relationship, with the elector feeling that the potential survivors are too entangled in religious or cultural norms to see beyond to the inexorable distress of terminal pain or acute mental illness. "Why can't she see how awful my life is? I can't live and endure the pain just for her sake," or just for the sake of faith or just for the sake of convention. Often potential survivors (Prado's term for those living with the elector's decision to die that has not yet been acted upon) are shaped by outside forces to reject suicide or assisted suicide and cannot see beyond their conditioned views to the actual, specific situation the elector finds herself confronting. Potential survivors, in the midst of the debate about choices, may realize that they are going to lose a loved one either way—it may be in a few days, a few weeks or a few months—and that fighting the voluntary choice to die is simply another form of denial. Listening carefully to the pain of the sufferer may help the survivor realize the extent of the suffering involved and help him muster the courage to let go because his loved one does not deserve the pain. In the elector's position we may have made a similar choice. Ironically, love can blind us to another's pain.

•　　•　　•

I needed more than a philosopher's perspective on these questions. I wanted to speak to real, live people who work in the trenches with these decisions, rather than read the small print of academic tracts alone. I turned to Elliot, who has been a psychiatrist for almost thirty years; he began a fascinating study with children who lost parents at a very young age, and his research spun into much more work on death and bereavement. Over his lengthy career, he moved from adult psychiatry to working with children because he wanted the range of clinical variety to satisfy his intellectual interests.

"I've always been interested in the emotional aspects of life and the workings of the brain," he said, because "you're not treating the chart, you're treating the person. This isn't about the disease. Because it's about the person, it's endlessly interesting."

Elliot believes that his career choice ultimately brought him into contact with incredibly meaningful work. "I'd never give it up for another specialty because it involves the deepest part of human existence. But you have to take care of your inner well-being and find ways to heal the wounds that it opens and regain your perspective and balance." Elliot understands that when you work closely with death and with the myriad ways that human beings become their own worst enemies, you have to find ways to salvage yourself. For Elliot, it's music. "For me, my family was an outlet, but music became a very wonderful way to be in touch with some very deep, deep and closed-off emotional pain and awareness of life that came from seeing the suffering that I was exposed to."

The exposure to deep pain began when Elliot did a research fellowship on the development and pathology of emotional awareness and the ability to read and express emotion in young children. He wanted to study early childhood depression and worked under a very

well-known researcher who told him that we don't know what the clinical criteria really are in young children. He recommended that Elliot
start his research with children who had a clear depressogenic event, an
event that would be likely to cause depression. He began with a study of
three- to six-year-olds who had recently lost a mother or a father. Over
the years, he increasingly saw patients who were grieving a loss or who
suffered deep depression and wanted to take their own lives. While he
feels blessed never to have had one of his own long-term patients take
his or her own life, he often sees families who are gripped by loss due to
a suicide. Sometimes recovery takes years; sometimes it never happens.

When I questioned Elliot about free will in the case of suicide, he
hesitated before answering:

> It's pretty rare that a psychiatric suicide is done with free will in the
> full sense of the word. There are many who do it on impulse and have
> not planned it. More often there is some level of planning; sometimes
> it's been revealed and sometimes it's not. Many who plan it and arrive
> at the decision are not doing it of their free will. The power of the
> brain is such that one has altered judgment, and can alter thought
> processes. The person who is delusional or has fixed, unshakable be-
> liefs is not making a decision shaped by reality. What that says is that
> the brain is so powerful that people's thought processes and thought
> content is affected by their neurobiology. The decision-making pro-
> cess when someone feels agitated, hopeless and helpless causes a
> person to draw conclusions that they wouldn't ordinarily arrive at in a
> state of health.

Ideally, if therapy and medications work, the patient can arrive at a
more balanced state of health and reconsider the impact of her decision. But sometimes she never regains that balance.

I asked Elliot if he can maintain professional neutrality in such cases. He said that he can and that he must in order to be effective, but that "when the family leaves my office I feel heartbroken and scared. I am very, very aware of how powerful the brain is and how easily it can turn on you and how quickly a person can become very different from themselves and be taken over by the demons of mental illness."

Elliot describes the fragility and malleability of the brain and how aware he is of it when he has difficult cases. Over time, he has come to recognize that there are many different aspects of intervention with families of suicide electors, an important part of which is helping the family understand suicide as a symptom of an illness. In most instances, he claims, there's been an effort to treat the illness, but sometimes the process was so quick and ferocious that there wasn't time to intervene or the person was too secretive or ashamed or didn't allow him- or herself to be adequately treated. Elliot has to help the family understand mental illness, retreat from self-blame and then help mitigate the anger toward the deceased. Only after that can the family turn toward grieving the loss.

> They can't do that beforehand because the suicide is such an overwhelming barrier; it's so fraught with complicated emotions they don't get to acknowledge, accept and work on their sadness and loss. I'm helping them get to the point where they can grieve.

Everyone needs an opportunity to mourn and experience loss. In suicide and assisted suicide cases, there is often a great deal of unarticulated anger that stands in the way of mourning. Anger is self-generative, and it can remain churning in the system for decades as a substitute for sadness. What Elliot was doing was allowing families to feel sadness, giving them permission to grieve by letting go of anger and other emotions that cloud sadness and make it hard to get to. Finding sadness is like finding a small, hidden door in a large, imposing house. But Elliot helped me understand the importance of arriving at that door, standing in front of it and opening it up to let the grieving begin.

Elliot shared the complexity of suicide for survivors and why closure is so hard to come by. The elector may have a happier ending than the life he or she was living, but the grief that pools for survivors seems beyond measure.

And then I spoke with Darin, who does not believe in closure at all. Darin has a recurrent dream—nightmare, actually—and then it goes. But it always comes back, jumping up at him when least expected. Darin's wound will find no closure because twenty-three years ago he hit a schoolmate who had swerved into the path of his car; most likely it was a death wish. Just that morning, she had written about how she wanted to take her own life but instead had someone else do the job. Darin did not know her personally well enough to grieve. Instead, he grieves, on some level, for himself, for the loss of life that he experienced because he did this and cannot fully live with himself.

It was a few weeks before his high-school graduation. Darin was eighteen years old and driving his car in late spring with friends on Long Island, when a schoolmate cycling with a friend swerved her bike into his car and died. Darin was exonerated of any charges; the girl had intentionally cycled into Darin's car. The police report freed him of blame, and her parents forgave him. But he has a rough time forgiving himself, even decades later. He shared some research with me on post-traumatic stress syndrome after drivers hit and kill others. If you know you were in the wrong, you experience less PTS than if you hit someone unintentionally. "It just seems so counterintuitive," he tells me, "but I guess it's true." When others punish you, you can accept the blame, having paid a price. No one found fault with Darin, so he keeps finding fault with himself. "I'd done something incalculably big, and here I was, still alive."

Darin wonders if he had been a better driver, say a Mario Andretti, would she have been spared? And then he reminds himself that in the what-if game we often play, it doesn't matter. He hit her. He was not someone else.

Darin chose to tell his story to the world to take the weight of it outside of himself. He wrote a memoir called *Half a Life*. A novelist who had published books with major presses, Darin decided this time to go with a small publishing house because he was, in essence, doing this for himself. It wasn't important for him to get the kind of exposure he needed to build a career. "It was not fun to write, but it was very cathartic. It was easier to write than to carry around with me." He compares it to complicated grief-disorder therapy, a form of healing where the person suffering speaks his or her travails into a recording device and then plays it back every day, putting the tragedy into some kind of manageable time allotment rather than having it spill over everything all the time. "People think the reason it's effective is because you can turn the tape off. I think it works because you can speak it aloud. When you make a story about it, what comes first and what comes next, you have some degree of control over it." He compares writing the book to AA: it's like getting up in front of a room full of strangers and telling them something that is difficult. "I have spent a year and a half building the scab up. Talking about it so much has made it easier to deal with it. It works against denial."

But writing the book and outing himself was only a limited help. For years after the accident he wondered at what point in dating women should he tell them. At job interviews, he asked himself the same question. After the book came out, he had to tell and retell the story at book signings and at schools. "I don't believe in closure," Darin tells me. Sometimes we call an act, a discussion or an event a

closure when it is a false label we offer ourselves because we have decided to move on, regardless of what we really feel. "I need closure,"
we might say to others, but is closure ever really on offer? Is it ever
truly possible to tie a problem or an emotional itch into a nice bow
and send it off into the past and never think about it again? We are
humans, not robots. We live through time and experiences, and they
come back to us, perhaps visiting us in a different way and without
the intensity of their initial shock, pain or joy. But they are there, and
for some, these events play themselves back to us like a looping video
we wish we could turn off, but we cannot. It made me recall Rumi's
poem "The Guest House," where our emotions visit us, and we decide how and if we will greet them:

> *This human being is a guest house.*
> *Every morning a new arrival.*
> *A joy, a depression, a meanness,*
> *Some momentary awareness comes*
> *As an unexpected visitor.*
> *Welcome and entertain them all.*
> *Even if they're a crowd of sorrows*
> *Who violently sweep your house*
> *Empty of its furniture,*
> *Still, treat each guest honorably.*
> *He may be clearing you out*
> *For some new delight.*
> *The dark thought, the shame, the malice,*
> *Meet them at the door laughing,*
> *And invite them in.*
> *Be grateful for whoever comes,*
> *Because each has been sent*
> *As a guide from beyond.*

Darin had been entertaining an unwanted guest for a really long time. But he did not rush to send this guest away. Darin acknowledges now that the accident informs his life and that it was very difficult, but that the difficulty has softened over time. He thinks about it often but says that he would not want to think about it less because it would make him less human. "At the end of the day, no matter if you forgive yourself, the fact is that you killed someone."

We spoke about his need for forgiveness. Although the girl's parents initially forgave him, they were later encouraged to sue him, which undermined any acceptance of Darin's contrition. When they sued him, he was a mess. "The financial nervousness was real. I was an eighteen-year-old kid with no money in the bank, and they were suing me for millions of dollars, so I knew that they hadn't really forgiven me." Her mother once said to him, close to the accident, that because he was alive, he now needed to live for two, placing another burden on Darin's weak shoulders. "I went through my twenties hoping that they would someday forgive me, even though I knew intellectually it wasn't my fault."

I don't need their forgiveness because I don't need to seek forgiveness from people I never want to talk to again. Even though I feel terrible about what they went through and don't blame them for suing me because I don't know how hard it is to lose a child, I don't think it was morally healthy to require forgiveness from them when what I really needed was the ability to accept emotionally what I knew intellectually. You never get over something like this fully. Closure implies that it's gone. You close this chapter and move on to the next chapter. I don't think life is structured in that way.

After he speaks about the accident in public, he always feels a little lighter. And perhaps he has created that for his audience as well. He told me that the book had much more universal appeal than he expected, because there are so many people managing guilt for crimes they did not commit, guilt without culpability, guilt without reason. He could write a whole book based on the letters and e-mails he received, like the one from a woman whose twin brother was born with a birth defect. She has spent her whole life feeling guilty for being healthy.

Darin needed self-forgiveness but could not grant it. He has been contacted by psychologists who ask him why he is not angry at the girl for cycling into his car and causing him years of insecurity and doubt. But Darin is not harboring anger. "How could I be angry at her? I'm alive, and she's not." He told me that he feels he is in a healthy place right now emotionally about the accident. I ask him if he ever visited the grave, and he confesses that when he was eighteen he thought about it but was not brave enough. He has gone back to the site of the accident, but it did not generate the pain he anticipated. I ask him if he could visit the gravesite now and ask forgiveness of her. He is not sure. He thinks so. Her friends have contacted him over the years, and one asked him to speak a few months ago at the high school in which she teaches. He asked the teacher if she had the address of the cemetery and took it. "Maybe I'm not in as healthy a place as I thought because I've had the address for a few months and haven't gone." He is not sure what he would say. There is no script for tombstone conversations.

Darin says he's sorry to her on occasion, what he thinks of as a silent acknowledgment of the accident. Years ago, he claims he was "consumed by immature selfishness—as often as I said 'sorry' to her I would think about my own future. How can I mitigate the effect of this and move on? There were times when I was apologizing and times when I was pretending this had no effect on me." The effects on him to this day are more clear with hindsight. "I am very uncomfortable with people thinking I did something bad, especially if I don't think I did it. I am more sensitive to criticism than most others. Maybe I am more desirous of approval and good will from people. And there are certain TV shows I have trouble watching; if it's a story where someone is accused of doing something he didn't do, I get very uncomfortable. I squirm or leave the room. I turn off the TV. I say 'sorry' more than I have to. I go far out of my way to avoid conflict. I certainly need forgiveness more than most people." Rumi's guest stays. "I have to live with this all the time. How can we know we are not at fault and yet still feel at fault? I know these things are never fully over. It's forever."

The wound closes up a little but not altogether.


We all know people who have taken their own lives. We know the survivors. They are the walking wounded who live their lives as one big question mark, who have trouble waking up because they cannot answer the question "Why?" that haunts them because of the death of a parent or a child or a friend. "It's forever." Like in Alice Sebold's novel *The Lovely Bones*, I somehow imagine the dead through suicide walking the world of the living and watching how their deaths ate away at those they loved and at people they never thought would be so profoundly affected by their absence. I wonder: if they could have seen the irreparable warping of other lives that their deaths cost, would they have done it? To me, suicide is not Seneca's ultimate act of freedom. Except as a choice between painful terminal illness and death, suicide is an act of ultimate cowardice, of selfishness, of narcissism, even when it cannot be helped. The beautiful deaths that people shared with me were beautiful for the dying *and* the surviving. Suicide is not a happy death, not for the elector or the survivors. At most, it may be a relief for the elector.

Perhaps I believe too strongly, with an almost irrational conviction, in the power of life and the possibility of reinvention. I witness our capacity to change every day. I see it in my friends, my students, my children. I watch it in myself. I see how the change in circumstances alters reality for good and bad and how events in our lives that we could never anticipate change us for the better. I see the impact of medicine to manage and sometimes cure mental illness and depression, and I feel anger and disappointment when people who need these drugs stop taking them and, as a result, make poor judgments that are often life-threatening.

If, as Heraclitus said, you can never step into the same river twice, then every moment becomes pregnant with chance. The person who ends it all tells himself that every day that follows will look like every day that passed, and for that it is not worth living. But I see each day ahead as unlike every other day I've ever lived, and I wonder how anyone can ever give up on that possibility.

## Chapter Five

# Denial, Resignation, Inspiration

Dying is easy. Parking is hard. The witticism belongs to humorist Art Buchwald, who, as it happens, had a lot to say about death. At the age of eighty he had severe kidney problems and had already lost a leg. His doctors wanted him to undergo dialysis. He figured he'd had a good, long life and didn't want to end it with physical suffering. Welcoming death was the noblest option at this point. He said goodbye in his long-running *Washington Post* column and checked into the Community Hospice program in Washington, D.C. In the great way that doctors let you know how long you have left, Buchwald was told he had three more weeks until D-day. Friends and glitterati came to visit and say goodbye. Buchwald claimed that he loved every minute of it. In dialysis, he would have disappeared. In hospice, he became a celebrity. "Hey, Buchwald's dying in a hospice. Go over there. It could be a good story."[1] He ridiculed the way that people never know what to say to a dying person. "You look great!" just didn't work.

After two months in hospice, Buchwald's doctors presented him with a medical mystery; his kidneys actually *stopped* failing, and, like a prisoner whose execution is suddenly stayed, he got to leave hospice and squeeze out one more book. *Too Soon to Say Goodbye*, the title of the book, was also the title of a song that his friend Carly Simon wrote for him when he announced to the world that he was entering hospice care. Buchwald called himself the born-again columnist. The little extra bonus time gave him the chance to make everyone laugh again, but this time with the added advantage of feeling deeply blessed for the reprieve.

In my quest for a better death, I came to disagree with Buchwald. Dying and parking have more in common than you think. Both involve unknowns. Both are irritating. Both eat up time that could otherwise be better spent. Both make us unhappy. Both can be costly. And you may be better at this than I am, but in my case both involve skills that require greater mastery than I currently have. And, if I'm not mistaken, cemeteries look like they involve a lot of parallel parking.

Buchwald's encounter with imminent death may have given him some unexpected gifts. But how does that help us, those of us who aren't slated to meet the scythe of death anytime soon but who realize it could happen at any time? Buchwald's death was not like my cousin Alyssa's death. It was hardly sudden, and then for a while, it wasn't at all. It gave him time, enough time to write a book. It also gave him time to go through the three stages mentioned in the Preface: denial, resignation and inspiration. The end of his life ended up being almost indescribably beautiful, not only because he was given a reprieve from death—a reprieve does not mean it isn't going to happen, only that it's delayed—but because he was able to embrace it and share it lovingly with others. He had reached the stage of inspiration, but to get there he had to go through the previous stages of denial and resignation.

Of course, none of us knows when our time will arrive to begin preparing for this inspirational last season. As it says in the book of Psalms: "His breath departs; he returns to the dust; on that day his plans come to nothing."[2] Whatever you wanted to achieve in this brief lifetime might come to an abrupt, unpleasant and unanticipated end. Your grand plans may come to nothing. If we could only know the ETA of the angel of death, we might, like Buchwald, be able to make some satisfying plans, check off a few more things on the bucket list and check into a closing period of blessing and gratitude. If we could study death from this vantage point, perhaps we would feel more mastery over it.

As my search for the better death continued, I learned that the closest approximation we have of our ETA is actually only a click away. If you really want to know how long you have left, try the mortality calculator, otherwise known as the death clock. Just Google it or try the iPod app. Originally conceived by life insurance brokers, the death clock requires you to put in your age, gender, and health status, and then it spits back a number that is the average time you have left. You need to plug in your birthdate, your weight and height for your body-mass index, your country, whether you're a smoker, your regular alcohol consumption, your general outlook on life—not taking into account, of course, random accidents, great genes, natural disasters, sickness and other indices beyond calculation. All of these factors affect death rates. These websites usually offer a mortality stopwatch that begins the countdown as soon as it finishes calculating your remaining years. It's a thought-provoking addition to your morning jog.

I wanted to see how consistent these clocks are with one another, so I put my vitals into a few different calculators. According to one, my last day is January 3, 2062. Right now I have a whopping 1,602,075,228 seconds left. As I type that number dwindles. I'm going to type more quickly. That date is not too bad, but I would love a little more time. Did my outlook on life make a difference? It did. Being an optimist bought me six more years than the average pessimist with the same body-mass index. As I always suspected, my happy demeanor has paid off.

Another calculator computed my last day as Monday, December 27, 2049. While I do like the feature of knowing what day of the week I'm going to go, I never thought it would be a Monday, and I wanted to die on an even year or maybe rounded out to 2050. Mondays are depressing; I'm holding out for the weekend. I'm also not willing to give up thirteen extra years, so I'm sticking with the first website.

I recently showed the death calculator to a relative in his forties who is notoriously late for everything. I naively thought that if he knew how much time he had left, he'd have more of an incentive to get to places on time. At first he rebuffed me, but then he put in the requested information. A few seconds later "23 YEARS LEFT" flashed up on the screen in large Roman characters, right beneath his body-mass index and the unsolicited state of his health: "You are overweight." Behind this already frightening table of facts was a large, yellow glowing skeleton. Okay. So it wasn't such a good idea.

Having used the maudlin stopwatch for a few days to see if anything would change in my life, I began to find this way of measuring time frustrating to say the least. I now had to wonder not only if I had enough time to complete a small project before doing carpool, I also had to calculate how many carpools I might have until the end of it all. Unfortunately, it was still thousands. The numbers were alarming. I found myself wondering not how to pack my days with more ambitious plans and manage the pressure of my now urgent wish list but also how to outlive the average lifespan in my category. Most of these calculators expect that reaction and conveniently take you to links like "How to Delay Death." Click on it and it takes you to a health calculator and various advertisements for vitamins, treadmills and other health products. At this point, if they advertised unicorn juice and fairy dust from the elixir of life, I'd probably buy it just to up my numbers.

I realized that the death clock was not helping me overcome the fear of death, it was actually escalating it. And I could imagine that it would only make elderly people more nervous, paralyzing them from doing anything. If someone had only, say, 220 days left on the calculator, would he take up the ukulele? Not likely. What does the calculator do if you run past the allotted time? I wondered about these questions, but I learned my lesson with my always-tardy relative. I won't be sharing this particular application with anybody else any time soon.

Irritating though it was, the death calculator does work as a dash of sobriety in the happy punch our culture loves to drink. Naturally, there are other ways to accomplish this goal. A colleague of mine, for example, has his own coffin. He lies in it occasionally to anticipate the experience of death and remind himself of his mortality. It would seem an effective, if not somewhat gruesome, technique for making more out of life. When he gets up from that coffin, he must feel pressure to do something really meaningful, or maybe he hugs his wife and children a little tighter. Maybe he wonders if the coffin is comfortable enough for an eternal rest so he test drives it on occasion to make sure the necessary adjustments are made.

I don't have the ideal architectural space in my house for a coffin right now, but I can only imagine how meaningful life would be if I used both the death calculator feature on my computer *and* the coffin. The combination is unbeatable for inspiring productivity. Maybe I can borrow the coffin for the days I have writers' block.

• • •

I've learned to joke about death to avoid the somber confrontation with it that happens so often. But I've also learned that joking about death helps us anticipate some of its more frightening aspects in a safe, manageable way. Joking about death is, in a strange way, a form of denial but also a subtle way we study death, if you believe what the philosopher Ludwig Wittgenstein said: "A serious and good philosophical work could be written consisting entirely of jokes." We all know what the jokes mask, what we're afraid of: the sudden discovery of a growth, a physical malady that mushrooms into something uncontrollable and life-threatening. The special plans we have for ourselves dissipate in an instant and are replaced with gruesome premonitions of not being here, of not living.

My friend Christine, a lapsed Catholic, just went through that nightmare with her husband, Dennis. Eleven months after a seemingly innocuous visit to the doctor, Dennis was dead. Her nightmare is our nightmare. The difference is that she lived it. Christine and Dennis plodded through each stage of loss at an accelerated rate. They fought reality at the stage of denial. They slowly surrendered to reality at the stage of resignation. Then they prepared for the stage of inspiration, and it culminated in a tender, loving death.

Christine is dumbfounded by the radical change in her life but also strong enough to be able to smile at death now. At times, she looks beyond me when we talk. "I still think it's someone else," Christine says as she shakes her head back and forth in disbelief.

It happened to someone else. Not us. Other people also said that to me when we started telling people that Dennis had stage-four cancer.

I know what they were thinking: "If it happened to them, it could happen to us. I know them. They're not the cancer type."

What, I wondered, was the cancer type?

Christine got to know Dennis when she was in college and he was in graduate school for engineering. His best friend was her dorm neighbor, and he kept talking about this guy Dennis, and she finally said to her roommate, "Who is this Dennis?" She received her answer when he came to visit. "He's pretty cute. Smart, funny. When he walked up the stairs, I thought, *That's it. That's the guy I'm going to marry*. Remember, though, I was twenty-one and stupid." It was the early 1970s, and Christine described herself as a scruffy, braid-wearing kid in jeans who suddenly decided to clean herself up for the stranger on the stairs. "I took a shower, took out the braid and put on a nice dress, and then Dennis talked to me." They got married when Christine was twenty-two. "We were married for forty-two years."

In their last year of marriage, Christine and Dennis made a wedding for their first son, Todd: "It was really one of the happiest days of our lives, like a scene from *Goodbye, Columbus*. It was just wonderfully embracing. There was no tension. And then our son went on his honeymoon. Dennis was always overtly concerned about his health, and he didn't feel well. Two weeks after the wedding, Dennis went to the doctor." Dennis was a successful engineer with many international projects who did a lot of work in Africa and was scheduled to go there in a few days' time; his doctor thought it might be an ulcer and sent him off to get an endoscopy. The doctor's office was on a street with many medical practices so Christine, ever efficient, dropped Dennis off and then went to her ophthalmologist down the street. Oddly, as she was waiting in her doctor's office, she felt nervous and began to sweat. Something was not right; Christine told the receptionist that she was leaving just as she got a call from Dennis's nurse telling her to come to the doctor's office directly. She walked into the room, and the doctor said, "I think I see a cancer. It's small. It probably hasn't spread. We'll take off part of his stomach, and it'll be nothing." Christine was winded but had the presence of mind to ask if they could have more tests done immediately. After days of moving in and out of medical offices, they discovered the grim news: Dennis had late-stage cancer, and it was more serious than anyone ever imagined. Christine had not prayed in a long time. She wondered where Jesus was in her life now. Was this some big divine test? Should she get down on her knees?

In those first weeks, everyone played the numbers game: "One doctor said there was a 30 percent survival rate. Someone else said 70 percent. Then we heard 90 percent." They did not know what to believe. "I told myself," Christine said pensively, "that I could live like this for five years, a reduced quality of life. We'd just slow everything down and lead a more sedentary lifestyle. If I had to go with Dennis twice a week to doctors' offices, I was prepared. I could do that. I'm a realist. We started making calls on the way home. We called the kids."

They began to look for a doctor to shepherd them through the ugly dance of cancer now that they had to learn the steps.

Christine and I talked about what she and Dennis were looking for in their doctor hunt. They were seeking skill and experience, and someone who was not going to tell them what they wanted to hear but what they had to do. They wanted as much information as they could get. The internet has made this task easier but also more potentially frightening, since patients and their families soon go into information saturation and overload. Christine and Dennis were well connected, between her family and his engineering firm. Christine is well organized. She's a list maker, and she does her homework. "Dennis hated all my lists because I usually had things on them for him to do, but I didn't want to be afraid, I wanted to solve the problem. I went into full administrative mode: planning, programming, getting all the paperwork done. That's how I deal with things." She was not, however, willing to prepare for Dennis's demise. As practical as she is, this piece of information was not acceptable. Yet.

Christine translated her fear into intense pragmatism and realized, with all the different percentages of success rates being tossed about, that the arbitrariness might be a result of their doctors being, on some level, just as willing to entertain denial as their patients. Christine was not accusing anyone of lying, but she needed more confidence, and it took weeks to find.

Doctors, just like patients, buy into and sell false hope when it comes to dying. Studying death when it sits at your door requires pressuring the experts. Christine did not want false assurances. She wanted reality, cold and brutal as it was, but she also wanted a reality that Dennis was a part of, a future together. Doctors and nurses in an emergency department will often go through the motions of saving the patient, especially a child or a young person, even when they know upon arrival at the hospital that the patient is close to death and beyond saving. It seems counterintuitive, a medical farce. But far from being a waste of staff time and resources, such a "show" gives the family the feeling that the medical team did as much as they could do, although much, if not all, of it may have been medically unnecessary. It smoothes the transition from shock and horror to understanding and initial acceptance. Sherwin Nuland, citing the late William Bean, a professor of medicine at the University of Iowa, calls such behaviors

the busy paraphernalia of scientific medicine, keeping a vague shadow of life flickering when all hope is gone. This may lead to the most extravagant and ridiculous maneuvers aimed at keeping extant certain representative traces of life, while final and complete death is temporarily frustrated or thwarted.[3]

Nuland also identifies a contrasting moment, the time when physicians, no longer able to help their patients, disappear both emotionally and often physically from their patients, and how this abandonment also contributes to an unhappy ending, an end characterized by shock, anguish and a miserable lack of preparedness. In a survey of medical literature, Nuland concludes that the medical profession attracts people who fear failure and who often have particularly high anxiety about death. The dying patient then becomes the manifestation of weakness and failure, someone to avoid.[4]

Nuland's honesty makes me wonder how doctors contribute to dying well or dying miserably. By confronting their own personal challenges and overcoming the perceived weakness of failure, they can be emotionally and physically engaged with a patient until the very end of life, helping the dying and their families learn the facts so they can face their fears. Admitting defeat is a nod to nature, and to the extent that doctors can offer humility in the face of death, they may be able to help their patients' family and friends come to terms with the inevitable.

My friends Jack and Adele were never prepared to have that conversation with Adele's doctors. She had breast cancer a few years ago and five good years of remission. But the cancer returned just when they assumed they had beaten it, and this time it was ferocious. Adele went in and out of the hospital, but she acted to her three girls and her friends as if nothing was wrong. She forbade anyone to talk about it, and the circle of those around her indulged Adele, knowing it would be the last game she ever played. Adele's hair fell out, she lost weight.

She lay listless as relatives from near and far came to speak with her. The word "death" was not mentioned. Because no one talked about death with Adele, and Jack would never speak of it in her presence, Adele never said her goodbyes properly. She never dispensed the wisdom she had gained as a mother, wife and professional. She never wrote down her last wishes or her hopes for her three girls, none of whom have fully recovered from her death even years later. Her own sister, Joyce, traveled a distance to spend the last many weeks at her bedside. When I spoke with Joyce during those weeks she confessed that no one was ready for Adele's death, even though the moment was imminent. I asked if there was something she could do to get them to talk openly.

"Adele's refused the social worker's visit or any clergy. She won't let anyone in," Joyce said. "I'm terribly worried about the girls. She's so very stubborn. Can't she see the harm that this will do to the whole family?"

Adele could not see. And she refused to see through the bitter end. Part of me can't blame her. Nuland, as a physician who counsels honesty with younger doctors and patients, identifies this curse of denial with his own Aunt Rose: "We knew—she knew—we knew she knew—she knew we knew—and none of us would talk about it when we were all together. We kept the charade to the end."[5] If we are under the illusion that such a charade has redeeming qualities, Nuland immediately disabuses us: "Aunt Rose was deprived and so were we of the coming together that should have been when we might finally tell her what her life had given us. In this sense, my Aunt Rose died alone."[6] If we push off death's approach in conversation rather than talk about it, then we won't prepare ourselves or our loved ones for the very last day and the painful day after that. Kübler-Ross, however, believes that denial is a very important stage in facing death, and its significance should not be underestimated: "Denial functions as a buffer after unexpected, shocking news, allowing the patient to collect himself and, with time, mobilize other, less radical defenses."[7] She believes that this slowly gives way to acceptance, but only when the patient is ready to absorb the news. Christine and Dennis were not ready. It would take months to move from denial to resignation. Sometimes doctors begin the conversation too early, when the patient is not ready to integrate the reality of death into his or her life. When the patient can no longer face the facts and reverts to denial, Kübler-Ross believes that the doctor must terminate the conversation. But she also believes that physicians owe the dying and their families the opportunity for a constructive conversation while the patient is in relative health so that they can get their emotions and finances in order.

Ernest Becker grappled with this disavowal of endings in his Pulitzer Prize–winning book, *The Denial of Death*. Becker chiseled away at the blackest shadows of the human condition, writing that "the idea of death, the fear of it, haunts the human animal like nothing else; it is a mainspring of human activity—activity designed largely to avoid the fatality of death, to overcome it by denying in some way that it is the final destiny for man."[8] The pain, rawness and the ignominy of death, how we cope (or fail to cope), are always before us, yet we live in denial as a lifelong race to get away from it.

Only in our darker moments do we challenge our invincibility. I watched Christine on the periphery of that fear, knowing it existed but trying to push it away, the way that someone pushes on a door that we keep trying to close. The fears of musty closets and monsters under the bed give way as we age to far more demonic fears: rejection, unemployment, poverty, infidelity, divorce, loneliness, cancer, death. We face what the psalmist confronted when he wrote, "My heart is convulsed within me; terrors of death assail me. Fear and trembling invade me; I am clothed in horror."[9] We feel the tremors of this verse as it pulses within us. We recognize the difference between fear and trembling, with the semantic precision of Søren Kierkegaard: fear needs a direct object. We are afraid of *something*. Trembling seems to be a general state of horror, the type of dread that shakes every assumption we hold dear. Death can do that. It has that kind of sensory power over us. It is the drum that beats continuously in our brains, the cloud that hangs unwelcome over our best moments, the bitter aftertaste of all happiness.

Research in psychology offers a fascinating correlation: people with high self-esteem also have a heightened fear of death.[10] Those who think highly of themselves tend to have more anxiety about death, fearing that the end of selfhood will obliterate everything they have come to hold dear: themselves. Death paralyzes. It is the cessation of all activity and opportunity for self-actualization. The highly ambitious cannot face the fact that their ambitions may end unsatisfied.

But forget the death knell for a moment. Some people seem to have an inner clock that is more highly calibrated than others and manage to force more meaning out of time precisely because of their personal fear of death. Mark Twain said it best: "The fear of death follows from the fear of life. A man who lives fully is prepared to die at any time." The capacity to live in the present and maximize it softens the scare of not existing at all. If we really feared death, we would make sure to get it all in quickly before time runs out. The gift of death is that we don't know when it is, so we spend each day in exceptional states of love, generosity and sanctity because time matters so much.

Christine and Dennis initially experienced the denial that Nuland captures so well. Christine claimed she was a realist, but I reminded her of the first weeks of the diagnosis. They were both deniers. Dennis went from being a successful engineer to being a full-time patient in a flimsy hospital gown, what one greeting card calls an Oscar de la Venta. Dennis lost thirty pounds in ten days. Christine took a leave of absence from work. She told me she could think of little else but Dennis's next test. An avid reader, Christine told me that she could read only two pages of a novel per day. That was her distraction. I asked her if she wanted to talk about what she was going through emotionally. "I can't go there. I just can't go there. I'm not prepared to go there. It's not a good place. Right now, we're taking it one day at a time, and that's what we'll continue to do." Despite how rapidly her life changed, she still was not ready to talk about death. Again, they wanted cold, hard facts, but they wanted them to substantiate a particular conclusion: that Dennis was going to live.

Those who deny death pretend it's going to happen to someone, just not them. Human beings don't do death well because we are escape artists, every one. Despite all knowledge to the contrary, we are trapped in the irrational belief that we will not disappear. Kübler-Ross describes this as the basic knowledge that, "in our unconscious, death is never possible in regard to ourselves."[11] We ignore the ancient question posed in the Bible: "What man can live and not see death?"[12] We and those we love will do what no human beings have ever done before: live and love forever. As the Armenian-American author William Saroyan once famously wrote, "Everybody has got to die, but I always believed an exception would be made in my case." Kübler-Ross begins her chapter on denial with a story of a woman with a fatal illness who went from doctor to doctor, dismissing those who gave her a negative diagnosis, convinced that her X-rays had gotten mixed up as she shopped around for false hope.

Notoriety may only make this attitude worse. Debt-ridden and on his deathbed at the age of forty-six, Oscar Wilde famously said, "I am dying beyond my means!" In the confines of his home, wasting away in his last hours, he reputedly told a friend, "My wallpaper and

I are fighting a duel to the death. One of us has got to go." Despite the pain of what was likely a syphilitic condition, Wilde publicly made light of his last hours, using them as maudlin comic relief. But privately, he confided to a close friend that he was very frightened and he dreamed of death and of "supping with the dead." Knowing Wilde, his friend replied, "I am sure you were the life and soul of the party."

Wilde reminds us that at heart we are not really afraid of dying. We are afraid of never having lived. We are afraid of never making the big splash, the indent that shows we were here, that we mattered. We want full-blown lives of excitement and beauty and terror and drama. We tire of minivans and Happy Meals and gardening magazines. We dream big dreams far from suburbia but fail to actualize them. We ache for contentment. We yearn to feel that our lives are worthy of remembrance. We secretly want to take risks and buck convention and make a difference. *New York Times* columnist David Brooks asked people over seventy to write life-reports, essays on their lives about what went poorly and what went well. He found these reports addictive reading and shared some of the life advice that they offered. One of his conclusions: "*Lean toward risk*. It's trite, but apparently true. Many more seniors regret the risks they didn't take than regret the ones they did."[13] We ignore death only to avoid the larger question of its significance in crafting a life worth living, in taking the risks to make life thrilling. The British critic G. K. Chesterton captured it the way only British wryness can: "There are people who pray for eternal life and don't know what to do with themselves on a rainy Sunday." We ignore death as a way to convince ourselves that we can live forever, but then again, who *wants* to live forever?

For some years, a colleague at work was responsible for posting the list of events in our office each day in the elevator. She used to add a thoughtful quote underneath the schedule, and I always looked forward to it as a little snatch of meaning each morning. One day she posted the following quote: "If what you have doesn't make you happy, why will having more of it make you happier?" Initially I thought of this in relation to possessions. Then I began thinking of it in relation to time, because that seems more elusive than objects. We can replace objects, but we cannot recover lost time. If you're not using your time well right now, why should you want more of it? Why should you deserve more of it?

Why? Because even if we don't know how to live, we don't want to die. The Belgian poet and playwright Maurice Maeterlinck said of us, "All our knowledge merely helps us to die a more painful death than animals that know nothing." But I disagree. Ignorance about death is not bliss. It can have devastating and irrevocable consequences.

Christine told me that when she got past the denial, she was very afraid that Dennis would die. This fear of nonexistence was paralyzing, and it drove her to either distraction or hyperproductivity. The philosopher Bernard Schumacher writes in *Death and Mortality in Contemporary Philosophy* that such avoidance is only natural: "Meditation on death is avoided like the plague, because we prefer to occupy ourselves with things that are less lugubrious, and, one might add, less obscene. Death causes those who speak about it to shiver and to experience an uneasiness mingled with a fear of their own death or the death of a loved one; it is mentioned only in cloaked terms."[14] Out of fear, we use language that masks and sterilizes death and makes it seem less harsh and frightening. We "pass on" rather than "die" because passing makes it sound like we are moving from one lane to another on a long highway instead of parking indefinitely at the rest stop.

Mostly what irked Christine was thinking about Dennis's funeral. "I was so scared of a funeral, but the funeral was actually wonderful. The eulogies were uplifting. Dennis made almost no requests. He didn't care where he was buried. He just asked that a few people say nice things about him at the funeral." I didn't understand why the funeral, the part she feared most in the process, went from being a nightmare to being inspiring. "He wasn't there, so I didn't think . . ." Christine spoke with reserve, perhaps wondering if her words sounded strange. "I didn't think of him as the one in the box. I thought when they lowered him in the grave it would be devastating, but not for one minute did I think that he was in that box." So where did Christine think Dennis was? "He was close by."

"Where is Dennis now?"

"Now he is so far away. He's dead. He's moved far away."

When I spoke to Christine months later, this had changed for her. "Now I think he is very close again, and letting me know he is close," she said.

Dennis's movement in and out of her life after his death was strange, but undoubtedly real for Christine. Not superstitious or mystical by nature, she is not sure how to explain Dennis's presence, but it doesn't matter. She knows he is with her.


As I spoke to more and more people who had watched loved ones die, it became apparent that the death of a loved one fortified them in some profound, unspoken way. They thought they could not live through the death of someone they loved, and then magically they lived. Life was not the same. But they were stronger than they ever believed they could be. No longer only having to imagine fear but having lived through it, they woke up to a different self, a self that was less scared. "I can do anything now," I heard again and again. I heard

Christine, a strong woman with a healthy sense of humor, say that she did not think she could live if Dennis died, but she did.

After the first six months of treatment and visits, Christine and Dennis resigned themselves to the new life they had and the inescapable reality that Dennis was never going to live through his cancer. When he felt better, they traveled to Italy and to Africa. Taking off from work suddenly did not mean anything in the scale of things. They wanted to use the time allotted wisely and well. Ironically, Dennis, the one who was always scared of illness, was no longer afraid. He loved going to doctors' offices. "He loved the doctors and the nurses. He loved the attention. He loved feeling that there was something he could do to help move his condition along." Christine thought that Dennis would struggle with the new onslaught of people in his life and would want to be left alone, but she was wrong. He softened. Going for treatment was a joy for him," Christine reflected. "People cared, and he felt that something could be done. You don't see frail people walking around chemo centers. Those people are beyond chemo. I saw strong people, and Dennis saw them too." As his life neared its end, he told Christine and others that he only suffered one night in the whole process. Even with infections and complications, this man who, according to Christine, usually complained every day about some ache or pain, did not complain. If anything scared Dennis it was the fact that his sister had died five years earlier from pancreatic cancer. He felt afraid for his mother. He felt afraid for his sons. He was less afraid for Christine. He said to her: "You're beautiful. You're smart. You're funny. You'll have some money. You'll be okay."

The one night Dennis was scared and in pain was the Sunday

before he died. Before that, a surgeon had operated on his perforated colon and bought him what Christine called "ten more days of happiness." But when Dennis experienced more tumors and realized that the next operation was just going to delay the inevitable, he decided, with the family's support, to go gently into the dark night. He was on a costly experimental drug. Each day came with a price tag, and each day was running out. As Christine tells it, "The surgeon looked at all of us and said to Dennis, 'I could operate, but there are tumors all over your intestine, and I am not sure how you would last through the surgery. It's your decision.' We all looked at each other and said no. This is it." Christine and the boys began calling friends and family, and people began to fly in to say goodbye.

The last ten days of Dennis's life quickly turned from resignation to inspiration. Every day was beautiful in its own way.

People did express their regret about the situation, but Christine was not interested in their pity. Both their boys were in their mid- to late twenties. "I don't have young children. At least it's not a tragedy. When I said that, my friends tried to correct me—it *is* a tragedy—but I still don't think so." Dennis was only sixty-five when he died. It was hard not to see a life cut off by decades as a tragedy, but there was something she saw in Dennis that made her adamant that his death was not tragic. "My nephew is an Eastern healer. When my mother-in-law asked him after Dennis's death why her son was taken from her, he said that Dennis was in a very good place, and he was finished with what he had to do. He was done. You see, Dennis lived very intensely, and he loved his life. He loved his family. He was an amazing father. He was so involved in their lives, maybe even too involved. At the end, he tried to let go a little. The boys had to give him permission to go. They had to tell him that they were going to be okay. He loved me. He loved where he lived. When he died, he was ready."

Over Dennis's last ten days, he talked openly about his death. He understood its physical causes and its immense emotional potency, and he immersed himself in the spiritual life, asking deep questions and engaging in conversations around gratitude and forgiveness. Instead of ignoring death or fearing it, Dennis confronted it with curiosity, as if it were a puzzle, a tangram or a Zen koan. He denuded our language of its euphemisms and confronted death as one might greet a friend. He studied it, in a manner of speaking.

Maggie Callanan, a hospice nurse and author of several books on bringing comfort to those in their last days, made the case for studying death at a difficult time in her own life. When Callanan's father was dying, he pulled her aside to ask her one question that would frame his end: "There are classes in parenting, financial planning, maintaining your house, building a deck. Why aren't there how-to classes in dying? . . . I don't know how to do this. . . . I want to do it right. How can I be a good example to all of you in my dying? I have tried to live my life right, and now I want to die right."[15]

Imagine a how-to class on dying in your local community college. Would you take it? There actually are such classes. The study of death is called thanatology, and today you can actually do a degree in the subject at about a dozen universities in North America. *Time* magazine reported that in the early 1970s, there were only seventy American colleges that offered thanatology. In the past several decades, that number has multiplied, with universities recognizing that adding it to their course rosters is an important offering in academic maturation.

Callanan's father is not the only one to make the case for learning to do death better. The journalist Charles Krauthammer made a plea that we all learn the fine art of dying well, not heroically in the Greek sense but what Krauthammer calls a much lower standard: "just not dying badly."[16] For him dying badly involves death at the hands of a suicide bomber, or with the ignominy of Kitty Genovese who was stabbed repeatedly and ignored by her apartment neighbors, or dying on a day when your death becomes eclipsed by bigger news. He reminds us that Mother Teresa, one of the saints of contemporary life, died on the eve of Princess Di's funeral. It's not hard to imagine whose death got more coverage. For Krauthammer, a good death is merely not a bad death. Surely if we study how to die better we can strive for better than that. Krauthammer's death examples involve no act of control, and they offer us no inspiration.

In tracing the trajectory of Dennis's death, a few months after the funeral, Christine's initial denial and subsequent fear blossomed into all kinds of observations about death: what she learned about Dennis that she could only have learned when he was already gone, what she learned about her sons' resilience and what she learned about her own autonomy. All of this learning awaited her. It awaited her because she had moved from denial to resignation. She stopped fighting and started accepting.

Part of dying well is the decision to stop fighting when it's time to accept the reality of death. Society admires the hope and resoluteness of those who try everything to stop aging and terminal illness, from trying fad diets to alternative healing ceremonies. Some people's will to live is so strong that they will try virtually anything to live another day. The problem with the fighting spirit is that it can get in the way of acceptance and resignation, which allows people to do what they want to end their lives rather than in aggressive bouts of battling for more time. It ushers in the stage of resignation and helps prepare people for the stage of inspiration.

Marilyn Webb, author of *The Good Death*, introduces us to Judith, a woman who was diagnosed with cancer for the first time in her midthirties.[17] She and her husband, Moh, fought the cancer with every fiber of strength they had, even when it meant long commutes to the hospital and eventually relocating their home and two young children for better support. When the cancer resurfaced and brought with it a bad prognosis, Judith and Moh were prepared to ramp up their efforts. They went the medical route, but soon Judith found that she was tired of hospitals and medicines that were making her feel worse and weren't working.

Judith then made the careful decision to change her attitude and accept death. No more fighting. Just loving. As a result, her last months were exceptionally tender. Moh and their children savor the memory of a wife and mother who read stories, held their hands and told them repeatedly that she loved them. With the family's acceptance of the inevitable, Judith could finally let go of the struggle to stay alive and begin the ascent into death peacefully.

Once Christine accepted the reality of Dennis's condition, she was able to open herself up to the learning and expansiveness that resignation can bring. At the funeral and for the weeks immediately after, she received dozens of visits and letters. She had always seen Dennis as somewhat shy, wanting only to spend time at home with his sons and with her. But a more nuanced picture emerged after Dennis died. He was beloved in his company. He had helped many young engineers, making critical professional connections for them and mentoring them. "I'm where I am because of him," one wrote. Another flew in all the way from South Africa to be at the funeral, telling Christine that Dennis had saved his life because he had believed in him professionally at a time of great personal despair. Dennis was worried that his career was slipping even before he got sick, but whatever anxiety this caused him was not borne out by his colleagues. Where Christine saw him as more introverted, she learned that Dennis was far from it: "Apparently, he was always talking, talking, talking. He was genuinely entertaining. I didn't give him credit for the extent of the way he helped people. He had good friends. I feel a little bad that I didn't give him the credit. People loved him." The funeral was a comfort for Christine. She had worried that, having forsaken the church, she would not be welcome in her time of need, but that was hardly the case. The priest and church members embraced her with kindness, and it felt loving and right. She was so grateful. It put her back in touch with what she had loved most about religion: ritual, community, and friendship.

Because Christine was a planner, she was able to step outside of her situation and grow from it. She watched Dennis and learned from him. She told me that when it came to death, the last year of Dennis's life was indeed the most beautiful in their relationship. Dennis told each person who came to visit him during his last week what they meant to him. He said "I love you" constantly and also said "sorry" to everyone, especially family, close friends and people from work. Christine found herself leaving the hospital room because "I couldn't listen to all of it. Too personal. It was just too personal. Some of it I didn't agree with. Dennis would say how wonderful someone was, and I thought to myself, *They were okay, but they weren't that great.*"

As Christine was recounting this, she looked down, a cloud moving across her face.

"I went in for every one of his treatments and doctors' appointments," she said. "He needed me all the time. If we had any issues it was probably that. He thought he would have liked a more codependent life, but I wasn't that person." Christine needed her space but was concerned that she couldn't give Dennis all the support he needed. For the last year, however, the two were inseparable, and she felt that she had given him what he always wanted: herself. On the last day when he could properly speak, he told people who came to visit, "Christine is my life. She's everything." He then said to Christine privately, "You were exactly what I needed all along." And that was another last moment of inspiration for her because she always thought she had disappointed him by not giving enough of herself.

Jessica, a South African woman in her forties, talked about a similar shared moment after death between her mother, who died at sixty-five, and her father. Jessica's family lived on a sprawling farm in South Africa. Her mother told the family that when she died she wanted them to bury her ashes in a hole on the beach. What she did not say was that her doctors told her she was likely to die within only a few months. Her death was a shock to everyone, including her husband, who went alone to the seashore to bury her ashes. "We were all so shocked, but she had left a letter to my father—not for us—saying that he was the true love of her life and that if she could do her whole life all over again, she would do it all again with him. It was her last gift to him, really, just making sure he knew how much she loved him."

Dennis probably had a ministroke twelve hours before he died. His son asked him how he was doing at about nine o'clock in the morning, and he said, "I'm com—" and never finished the sentence. Those were the last words he spoke; he basically left his family with the solace that he died in comfort. Christine knew that it would be his last day, because the night before his stomach was bloated with fluids and his breathing had slowed down significantly. She knew it was only a matter of hours, that they had said what they wanted to say, and when he went to sleep, Christine decided to go to sleep as well. "I knew the next day was going to be very hard. I needed the sleep." But the next day was not as hard as she had imagined. The whole family was there: "We were all physically entangled on his bed with him when he died. It was really very beautiful."

There was that word again, "beautiful," and she said it with a softness in her eyes that confirmed she meant it. "There was nothing more I could have done. I did everything I could do. I was loving and devoted. I'm not usually a patient person, but somehow I had patience."

Christine does not obsess about the what-ifs that drive others crazy. She wants to live her life. She does not want to be permanently sad. In the first weeks she cried every day. "I cry a lot now but not every day. I don't feel sorry for myself, just for Dennis, even after his death." She also believes that her independence saved her from the fate of other women in her bereavement group. The other six women cried every time. They are finding it hard to get on with life without their husbands. "I thought to myself, *What am I doing here? I am not like these women, and I don't need more friends.*" So why *did* Christine go to these weekly meetings? "I told you: I'm a planner. I needed to check all the boxes: write thank-you notes, find a therapist, take care of the finances, speak to lawyers, join a bereavement group. It just seemed like what you were supposed to do." She said it like a studious kid out to get good grades, and now she could award herself an A for grieving. But this was part of studying death; it was going through the paces, doing what everyone did in the wake of death, doing what you were supposed to do.

"I actually became very fond of these women, and even though I thought that I didn't need more friends, we all need more friends." Among the group, she had lost her husband most recently when she joined this hospice-sponsored program. Dennis had been dead for two months when she became a member. The other women had lost husbands between three and twelve months prior. As they moved around the circle, women would complain of not being able to get out of bed or going to work and then crawling into bed when they came home. Their husbands had been perfect spouses. It seemed too much for Christine, and she said so publicly to them.

I know it's soon, but I'm up and ready. I can't say I'm not sad. But I never lived by myself. I can now hang a picture by myself. I can make plans and follow through with them. I can do what I want to do without checking in with someone else all the time. We were at peace with the process. It wasn't a surprise. Those were eleven of the best months of our lives. Dennis is dead now. I want a life.

The dam broke for everyone else. It gave permission for the other women to come forward with some very personal information. Some of their husbands had been struggling with addiction and others were not as loving as all the tears seemed to communicate. Christine gave everyone an outlet to speak more openly because she had done it. Maybe, she wondered out loud, they were following a script of what they were supposed to say, but it wasn't helping them. They weren't being authentic. They were betraying their real emotions, and it made death more ugly.

In the end, I realized that my friends who advised me against joining a group were probably right. I was choosing life, and the others were choosing depression. I left after a few sessions because I saw how different I was. You know what? No one bothered to call to ask if I was coming back. Maybe they didn't really want me there. Without me, they could go back to being depressed. I'm not saying my marriage was better—only that it might have been stronger.

Christine, in a way, stepped out of her experience, so that she could think about the impact death had on her: the way it shaped her priorities, the emotional and financial debris it left in its wake, the spiritual questions it percolated. And it made her understand that death can be beautiful and that life after those you love die can also be beautiful. The memories should not be cheapened by tacking the newly dead onto white burlap the way that butterflies are pinned down, labeled, and framed. Christine did not need the halo effect to love Dennis. She mourned the death of a good man but not a perfect man. His death was beautiful because, in the end, it was honest.

Christine studied death in the world's saddest classroom. She had the candor to look at her experience and describe it accurately. She was not following someone else's lines. She experienced denial and fear and resignation but then stepped right through them. She was following her mind and her heart, and it took her to places others were afraid to go: confessing that marriage is hard, that Dennis was difficult, that she enjoyed the new freedom of being alone without feeling that she was betraying Dennis by saying so. Even when she revisits the pain, she has found a place to put it. Her eleven-month trial may have been a test of endurance, but it has also taken her to a place of profound inspiration.

"I had a dream that he came back," Christine says wistfully about Dennis. "Why are you coming back now? How am I going to redo this sadness? I just had three terrible months without you," she bellowed to her late husband. Dennis was transparent in Christine's dream. "And then I realized that it was just me talking. He did not say any-thing." She pauses and then smiles. "At night I used to feel him hovering, always kindly. . . . He's not here now."

But Dennis will come back. He always does.

## Chapter Six

# A Different Bucket List

*He did the dishes,*
*Rubbed my feet,*
*Surprised me with tulips,*
*Took me to musicals even though he didn't like them,*
*Carried my bags while I did the shopping,*
*Held my hand.*

*He died of cancer four years ago.*

*Because he loved me,*
*I can stay in our home.*
*I can be here for our children.*
*I can afford to pay for their college education.*
*I can worry about the other things in life besides money.*

*He still loves me. And he still shows it.*

You may be moved to tears by this poem, but don't get too excited. It's actually the text of a magazine ad for life insurance sponsored by Life, a nonprofit life insurance company. I found an old *Newsweek* while scrounging for reading material at the gym to get me through the tedium of an elliptical workout. The poem was on the back cover. It made me pause. I never really saw life insurance as an expression of love, but there it was in black and white. I was meeting someone in a poem who did not leave unfinished business for his family to sort out at a time of grief and loss. This woman still felt the impact of her husband's love years after he died because he made financially responsible decisions to provide for her and their children. And this is one critical key to creating a happier ending: using time and money wisely to leave a legacy, to take care of whatever needs to be done so that you can leave the world in peace.

Not all of us get the death warning with enough time to tie everything up nicely in a bow, especially with sudden deaths, like Alyssa's. And it's not only personal finances that need tying up. It's the emotional odds and ends of a life that may need healing or repair. It's all the dreams and ambitions you held on to that may or may not get fulfilled. Death is more than the end of life. It is the annihilation of wishes and unrequited longings. It is the end of a conversation. It is final.

Viktor Frankl speaks famously of unfinished business as a rationale for survival in a book often cited as one of the most influential works of the twentieth century, *Man's Search for Meaning*. His central thesis, born out of both research and personal experience as a Holocaust survivor, is that the people who stand the greatest chance of survival are those who have goals to achieve, projects to finish, people to see. It matters less what the direct object of survival is—in other words, why someone needs to do a particular something; what matters is the drive to do *that* thing. Often people who have a reason to live or a sense of meaning in their lives can actually muster the ambition to survive circumstances that would easily swallow those without the same drive. It is not a guarantee, just a strong motivator.

This may explain one of the mind's many wonders. It seems that people can willfully prolong their lives to live for a special event or a special day. Both John Adams and Thomas Jefferson died on the fiftieth anniversary of July 4, 1776, the same day fifty years earlier when they both signed the Declaration of Independence. In 2008, Mitsuru Shimizu and Brett W. Pelham wrote a research paper, "Postponing a Date with the Grim Reaper: Ceremonial Events and Mortality," to determine if people could, indeed, postpone their deaths. They examined death records for millions of people using Social Security death index records over the past sixty-five years to determine whether or not people were more likely to die before or after a major holiday or special day: Thanksgiving, Christmas, New Year's Day or their birthdays. They concluded that people were more likely to die just after a holiday than before it.[1] This research was conducted again in Mexico to vitiate cultural factors associated with holidays, and the authors arrived at the same conclusion.[2] Researchers call these "ceremonial finish lines."


That's where the bucket list comes in. The term "bucket list" is most frequently associated with Rob Reiner's 2007 film of the same name, starring Jack Nicholson and Morgan Freeman as two old men performing crazy stunts as a way to spice up the last years of their lives. Based on the tender euphemism "to kick the bucket," the term floated around the media quite a bit before and after the movie.

Today, you can go on bucketlist.org and make your own list, tell the story of how you accomplished each goal and share your list with others as they share theirs with you. You can silently compete for who outdoes your fantasies and add an idea from someone else's list who may be more bold or courageous. The website does recommend that you keep your goals realistic. Don't write "Climb Everest" if you have arthritis and are afraid of heights. Keep it simple, like "Perfect my chili recipe" (actual last wish on the site). Chili might be really important to you, and you only get one lifetime to master the recipe.

I wanted to be impressed by what the users of this site wanted from life, so I scanned the lists that people shared. Some of them did not follow directions; they were extremely ambitious. Not surprisingly, next to "Goals Accomplished" was a big fat zero. Some lofty goals were sandwiched between goals that seemed ridiculous, like this list below:

- Break a world record
- Bake a cake for someone for no reason
- Get a guided tour of the Blizzard campus [a studio that designs video games]
- See the northern lights
- Ride a Segway
- Visit Socotra Island
- Go on a Bioluminescence Night Kayak Tour
- Touch a great white shark
- Take a hot air balloon ride
- See a tornado in real life
- Participate in La Tomatina in Spain
- Explore a coral reef
- Run the Boston Marathon
- Learn to skateboard

- Become a good swimmer
- Win an award/contest for my writing
- Get published
- Write a book
- Survive a bar fight (with no broken bones)

Break a world record. Bake a cake. Write a book. Survive a bar fight. Hmmm, which is most likely? I'm going for the cake. The guy who wrote this list actually checked off ten out of nineteen. Don't know if he's ever touched a shark, but he should probably leave that for last.

Imagine having to accelerate your bucket list or write it down urgently because you just learned that you had only six months left to live. How would that change things? What would you do with that time to take care of unfinished business? You might spend it in a state of inebriation on a Caribbean island. You might go to a monastery and pray or finally take that world tour you always dreamed of with your spouse.

One of the striking aspects of bucket lists is their orientation around activities, usually of the daring kind, instead of around emotional closures or the setting of spiritual or intellectual goals yet to be accomplished, except of the kitschy kind. With six months to live, how many people will really spend the time it would take to get "Read *War and Peace*" checked off? It's easier to skydive. Imagine a different list that didn't take a lot of time or money or bravado but required emotional maturity instead:

- Pray and really mean it
- Finish my graduate degree

- Say "sorry" to my dad
- Go on a silent retreat
- Take each of my kids on a separate trip
- Reconcile with my difficult sister
- Write a letter to my mother to say thanks for everything

This kind of unfinished business is a lot less glamorous but often much more significant. I began to realize just how significant when I met Betsy.

"I think it's very important to find out what's unfinished that makes you feel like you can't let go." Betsy is a registered nurse in the D.C. area who ran group discussions for the dying and their caretakers for ten years through the American Cancer Society. She listened to the stories of the dying, their pain, their dreams, and what she heard was that they needed closure in their relationships. "I could get the brother they haven't seen in twenty years and bring closure to all kinds of stuff. I could help families be present and not be afraid." Many people stand in awe of people like Betsy who work with the dying. *How does she do it,* I wondered, *and come home every night and eat dinner with her family?* But Betsy just doesn't think that way. She believes that helping people tie up the loose ends of their lives is one of the most important ways to help them on their journey toward death, and her generous heart wants to help improve that journey.

Betsy is no ordinary retired nurse. This former Roman Catholic nun is now a grandmother and an Episcopalian priest working for a Lutheran parish. Her life journey exposed her to many different angles of compassion, personally and professionally. Betsy's desire to help the dying came early, while she was still at nursing school. "It was a place and a time when you could really make a difference in people's lives and how their families survived." In her eyes, there is no more purposeful or rewarding work than what she does.

Betsy originally became a nurse because she was a Medical Mission sister for eight years, a nun whose calling was to be both a nurse and a sister in the Church. Raised in a Roman Catholic family of eight children, Betsy was the only one of six girls to become a nun. Her older sister wanted to be a nun but her father forbade it. I was intrigued by Betsy's story: why she became a nun, why she stopped and how she began working with the dying.

As a child, Betsy went to church every day for Mass and attended Catholic school. "The church lived in us as kids, and then when I became a nun, I lived in the church. It didn't seem so different." During her first three years as a nun, Betsy left her convent in Fox Chase, Pennsylvania, only once: to get her wisdom teeth out. Her life then was filled with prayer, study and physical work: tending the convent's farm, hauling manure for the convent's garden or cooking for a hundred and fifty. Betsy describes those years as the most liberating of her life.

> It was so empowering as a woman. I didn't think there was anything I couldn't do. No one told us otherwise. We all believed it. I loved every minute of being at the convent. The things I like most about myself were fed and nurtured there. The community was so affirming. The message in my all-female environment was that there is nothing you can't do. I wish I could have sent my daughter to a convent instead of college.

In the convent Betsy was with women who wanted to make a difference in the lives of others. These were women who knew about sacrifice and friendship and commitment.

As a young nun, Betsy studied theology and comparative religion. The changes of Vatican II were just taking effect, and the Church was in the process of becoming more open. The goal was no longer to baptize foreign babies but to address the social injustices of the world. The Medical Mission order was designed to provide medical care in parts of the world where medicine was hard to access, particularly for women. Many women in Third World countries would not see a male doctor or nurse and would sooner suffer death than bodily exposure. Betsy knew of stories where her sisters were given twenty-five dollars and sent to Africa or India to open a hospital and a nursing school.

> And they did it. They really did it. They took that twenty-five or fifty dollars and they created a medical system where there was none. That's who I wanted to be. I had such love for these women. They had such faith. They were so courageous. And we weren't going out to proselytize because God was in all religions.

Betsy knew she wanted to be a nun at age fifteen. She felt called to the Church but knew that her father would be against it. It was going to be, in her words, a battle. She prepared to tell her father when she was seventeen, over the Thanksgiving break. He was a traveling salesman and was not home often, so Betsy waited for a good time when she could have him alone. But when Thanksgiving approached, Betsy lost her chance. Her father had a major heart attack.

Because there were so many young children at home, Betsy's mother assigned her to stay in the hospital with her father for three weeks. She recalls those weeks with great fondness because she had her father all to herself. She could have adult conversations with him, and although she knew she couldn't bring up the subject of her calling because of his health, she was able to develop real closeness with him. It hurt all the more when he came home from the hospital and two days later had another heart attack that took his life. He was only sixty years old. "That was my introduction to major grief and loss, death and dying. When my father died it felt like my whole world shattered into a million little pieces. He died on the thirteenth of December, right before Christmas."

Every person's memory of someone they lose is different. After her father's death, Betsy realized that only those her own age could understand what it meant to lose a father so young. The uniqueness of each loss helped Betsy realize that caregivers and relatives need to be treated differently in their grieving. It's never a one-size-fits-all consolation.

The death of Betsy's father steeled her conviction to become a nun, but since her father had no life insurance, she put her plans on hold for a couple of months. Even with a married sister, there were still seven kids living at home. Her mother went back to work. It was a hard time, but slowly Betsy went ahead with her plans. In secret she contacted the convent community at Fox Chase and had all the mail sent to a friend so that it wouldn't arrive at her home address. Betsy only told her mother after she was accepted. After initial resistance, her mother accepted Betsy's plans. She then suspected that her own mother had wanted to be a nun but got married and had one child after another. "I think I was living a dream that she had at some point, so I was able to fulfill a wish that she had for herself."

Before she took her final vows, Betsy was sent to nursing school at the University of San Francisco for two years and then returned to the convent. She had been back only a week when a man showed up at the door with a newborn baby. His wife was sick (probably with postpartum depression), and he worked all night as a baker. No one could care for this baby, and the couple wanted the sisters to look after her for a little while until the family was back on their feet. The sister who took the baby was leaving for a thirty-day retreat the next day, so she put the baby in Betsy's care. That small, unexpected "package" changed Betsy's life. "It turned on every maternal fiber in my being. I played with her all night and carried her around in a laundry basket. It just broke my heart to give her back. It tore me apart." The parents did come back a few months later. By then Betsy knew that she could never take final vows in good conscience. "I couldn't say 'forever' anymore. My itch to have children was not going away." She renewed her vows just long enough to work in a foreign mission.

Betsy finished her training on the East Coast. She enjoyed psychiatric nursing and worked a full-time job in the field at Georgetown University for her senior year to support herself. She then went to Venezuela for a few weeks, believing that her calling was to work in medicine in Latin America. But her time in Latin America taught her something fundamental about psychiatric medicine: words are critical. Language is the way that people express their pain and their needs, and Betsy realized that in Latin America she could never succeed without the nuances and subtleties of the language. The work she was best suited to would bring her back to America.

When Betsy returned to the D.C. area to finish her degree, she met her husband, Ralph, a divorcé. Leaving the convent and marrying a divorcé felt like she was breaking every Catholic rule. But Betsy knew herself well and knew the path ahead; just as she once knew she needed to be a nun, she also knew that she had to leave. Her mother was devastated when she left the convent, as Betsy suspected she would be, but Betsy was finally going to fulfill her own dream of becoming a mother. She initially thought that all it took was reneging on her vows and getting married. But life was complicated for Betsy. She battled with infertility. Every direction she took had obstacles that she needed to navigate with delicacy. Her fifteen miscarriages became yet another way she understood misfortune, and she translated those experiences into emotional and empathic support for her patients. Expectation was buckled in with loss for her, again and again.

Leaving the convent was another type of bereavement Betsy had to negotiate. "I didn't want to let go of anything. I didn't want to lose these incredible women in my life. The bond is so strong. A Catholic is always a Catholic. If you were a Medical Mission sister, you are always a Medical Mission sister." She stays connected with her sisters, even twenty-five years later. Her order is represented in forty countries; it's not hard for Betsy to keep in touch with what she calls her spiritual home.

Somehow, Betsy knew she would be a mother one day. She and Ralph went together to her convent for a reunion weekend and ironically conceived their first child where once Betsy had taken her vows of celibacy. Finally, Betsy's own dreams of parenthood came true. But even as she stayed home to raise her children, Betsy did not let go of her concern for the dying. Betsy put her career on hold to raise her young children and ran groups as a volunteer for the dying and their families, as part of a group called Make the Day Count. She refers to herself as a mini-hospice before there was a hospice. Her board certification allowed her to do private practice, and this allowed her the space to develop professionally outside of the confines of a hospital. She spoke about care for the dying at a few churches and privately with some oncologists, and within a few months she had a full practice. She understood that the service she provided was nearly impossible to get anywhere else. "There was nothing else. People were desperate for someone to talk to."

Betsy's personal happiness as a mother and volunteer gave her the distance to face some unpleasant childhood trauma. She was finally able to understand some of the other losses that swirled around her home as she was growing up and how much sadness her mother bore (all of this became clear as Betsy was studying family systems).

At the time of my mother's birth, her own father was in jail for tax evasion. He was depressed and institutionalized. When I was born, there were six children under six. My mother's first child was a still-born, and then my brother died. . . . There was so much grief. When I left the convent, my mother never forgave me. My mother always told me what a perfect child I was, and it enraged me. If you have the per-fect child then your mother was a perfect mother. I married Ralph, who was divorced, and that was terrible for her. When she died at ninety-two, she sent a box of love letters to each of us. We found out that before she married my father, she was in love with a Protestant man but couldn't marry him because she was Catholic.

At the end, her mother suffered from severe osteoporosis and Alz-heimer's. Eventually she stopped eating and drinking because of the pain. She hadn't said a word in four days until right before she died, when she said, "It's so sad to lose a child." Betsy thought she meant Andy, her dead brother. But when she asked, "What child is that?" her mother replied, "Betsy."

Suddenly Betsy realized that she had broken the rules, but her mother had not. Betsy had done what her mother wanted to do but didn't. The way her mother died underscored the importance of help-ing others work out the emotional knots they've accumulated in life before the end takes away any possibility of resolution. Her mother had too much unfinished business and too many secrets. There was no hospice nursing to help her when Betsy lost her mother. Betsy knew that there was a better way to die.

Betsy believes that there are certain people who possess the art of healing, and that many people have this gift but are afraid to use it. "If you can remove your ego and really channel healing into someone else, then you can help people alleviate deep misery." Betsy prays for people on the other side of the world and believes that sending healing messages does bring some relief and repair to our broken world.

I asked Betsy to share the case that taught her the most about caring for the dying, and she talked about Joan. Joan had bone cancer; at that time, the only treatment was amputation. Joan already had one mechanical arm and she'd had her hip replaced. Doctors were literally cutting up her life bit by bit. But Joan was incredibly strong and determined. She had three teenagers, drove carpool with her prosthetics and did laundry. She wasn't looking for pity. Joan and Betsy decided to give talks together about dying to groups that needed it, and the two women got to know each other extremely well.

Over the course of giving talks about dying, they learned of a new experimental medication that Joan could take. It was dangerous, but it offered a slim chance of prolonging Joan's life, and she was a fighter. She wanted to live and keep going and would risk it all. She had the first treatment on Monday and was dead by Friday. She would never do carpool again. She would never do laundry again. Joan had given up a functional life for no life at all. At her funeral the church was packed. It was as big a funeral as Betsy had ever seen. Joan's daughter was angry. Where was this anger coming from? Betsy wondered. Everyone knew the experimental treatment was a risk. Her kids knew. Betsy took the daughter aside to speak to her, and she said, "Of the people here, besides you and your group, no one in this church called my mother, took her to lunch, asked how she was doing, asked if she needed any help."

It was a huge lesson for Betsy about the importance of community support. She believes that in order for people to "let go and let God," they need to be connected in at least four or five ways to a support community: friends, neighbors, parents of their kids' friends, faith community, work. "There are all kinds of reasons that people pull back. Some people just can't cope and so they draw back. I'm experiencing this with my husband's Alzheimer's right now. People at a cocktail party used to give someone with cancer a plastic cup instead of a glass because they were so afraid." Joan was coping so well with her responsibilities and was so extroverted that Betsy didn't realize until she died just how isolated Joan really was. The kids couldn't turn to any family friends for consolation because they had been abandoned by so many people while their mother was alive.

"That case changed the way I practiced. From that point on I realized that I cannot be the only support for someone who is dying." I asked Betsy what she does about this. "The first time I meet somebody I want to know if there are any friends that they're close to that they haven't heard from. One woman had a best friend who didn't call for a whole month when she found out she had cancer. If there's someone really important to you, I advise people to reach out. Just ask for practical help to stay connected."

Asking for help with specific tasks gives people who have difficulty coping with illness something to do that is within their reach. Reaching out may feel hard. We want our friends to come to our aid without the call for help. But ultimately people are wrapped up in their own lives, and they're not mind readers. It's sometimes hard to remember that friends are not omniscient, that they don't know all that we'd like or need them to do. This can cause a great deal of resentment, which, as Betsy testifies, can be just as toxic as illness to someone facing cancer or another disease. Through her years treating the dying, Betsy realized that there will be close friends you lose and strangers who will suddenly become very significant in your life.

Hearing Betsy reminisce about Joan reminded me of a question and answer I saw once in an advice column. Amy Dickinson, the woman behind "Dear Amy," was asked to share her wisdom with a woman named Morgan who visited a dying friend often. Morgan asked other friends to visit more often since their suffering friend was lonely. Some did. Some said they could not visit the dying friend at all, even though these "friends" had known her since childhood. It was simply too hard for them. Morgan was distressed. Amy responded that modern life has removed most of us from experiencing real suffering so we think that we can't cope because we may never have had to. Amy recommended that Morgan ask these friends to cook weekly meals or other specific tasks so that they could help in ways that made them feel comfortable. Reading this advice, I felt that Amy had given them a pass. Betsy would have insisted that they actually *see* their sick friend. Errands are important but not as important as genuine companionship.[3]

I felt validated a few weeks later when a woman wrote to Amy to question her judgment and directed her comments to Morgan: "To her 'friends' and anyone else in that situation, I'd have three simple words: suck it up."[4] The writer *was* that sick friend, and she complained bitterly that some of her lifelong friends could not be bothered to visit, call or send cards even though many lived only a few minutes away. She got the last word because she got better. Some of the friends who avoided her suddenly wanted her back in their lives.

> I really don't want these people in my life. I still have healing to do, and carrying around anger and resentment isn't healthy. I've recovered. But I don't think our friendships ever will.[5]

When Amy gave these friends an easy way out, she was thinking of their emotional needs rather than the needs of their sick friend. By not visiting, they had failed to accept their friend in the totality of her being.

In Jewish law, there is a special commandment to visit the sick. A famous rabbi was once asked if this commandment could be performed via the telephone. (Today the question would probably be "Can you text them instead?") He answered that when there are real geographic challenges or in the event that the patient does not want to be seen, the phone call suffices. Yet he cautioned that the commandment to visit the sick is not only for the benefit of the sick person. The visitor must see the person in his or her suffering because only after that face-to-face encounter will the visitor be truly empathetic when reciting prayers on his or her behalf. In other words, the visit does not only end when we see a sick person. The visual impact of seeing someone who is sick lodges those needs in our consciousness and helps us be more deliberate and thoughtful in our good wishes and deeds for the sick, something you just can't get from texting.

For Betsy, this form of denial is also what prevents unfinished business from getting done. Sometimes friends and family are in denial. Sometimes the dying are in denial. Betsy shared a story with me of a friend who died a couple of years ago. The friend was a former Medical Mission sister and a pediatrician who, like Betsy, eventually left the Church, got married and had three children. Sadly, her marriage ended in divorce. Some years later she was diagnosed with invasive colon and breast cancer. She was dying, but she would not allow Betsy or anyone else to talk about it. It was hard on Betsy because their lives followed such a similar trajectory. Her friend didn't want to go into hospice. "There is nothing more destructive than to see someone you love in horrible pain," Betsy reflects, "who doesn't want anyone to help her. This woman's children suffer now because they weren't able to talk through what was happening and get her the help she needed to die a better death."

Betsy's life and her work with the dying have taken a few strange turns. As her kids were growing up, she realized that, for her, the world of the spirit and the world of medicine needed to come together more holistically. She met her first female priest at a new church she and Ralph joined, and they became very good friends. Through that friendship, she had her next revelation: "I didn't have to make a choice between having a family and having a ministry." Betsy decided to become a priest. She started seminary when her son started high school and graduated when he did. She joined an urban ministry program.

> Eight of us were second- or third-career people. It was a real interfaith community. We traveled together each year looking at international ministries. We focused on inner-city stuff. My passion became ministering to homeless women. So many homeless people are abused by their church. I wanted to work with the victims, but that's not the normal role for Episcopal priests who run parishes.

The standing committee that grants ordination was very difficult to work with, and just when Betsy thought she would be ordained, her date for ordination was canceled because the church authorities decided not to ordain her. She was devastated. "They had decided not to ordain me after ten years of jumping through hoops. I railed at God. I was so angry. It was a huge expense for me and my family. What has this all been about?"

At that point, Betsy was finished even trying. She had words with God: "If You want this to happen, You're going to have to do some miracle working." And her miracle happened. Four hours after the cancellation of her ordination, she got a call from a woman whom she had met seven years earlier. She and her husband were the central ministers to the homeless in Washington, D.C. "She said she had wanted to contact me for years but couldn't remember my name. Suddenly she remembered that I had given her a book with my inscription and that helped her locate me. She told me that she and her husband were retiring and wanted to put my name in for the job. Was I interested?"

The job involved running a huge shelter for homeless women in a very run-down part of the city. Betsy told her about her ordination difficulties in the Episcopalian church, and the woman had a solution: "I'll make you a Lutheran." Betsy didn't care about the denomination because, in her eyes, it's all the same God.

> I had given up, and God parted the seas and made it happen. Someone once said to me, "Betsy, you want this too much." I never knew what that meant until that day. . . . It's really all God's work. God was waiting for me to give up, telling me not to try so hard. Don't try hard. Let Me be in charge so that you know it's about Me.

The next day Betsy spent the whole day in and out of interviews with the standing committee, and by the end of that day they accepted her. Betsy looked back on her life. She grew up a Roman Catholic, went to a Methodist convent, worked in a Jesuit hospital, had Episcopal training and, finally, a Lutheran ordination. For her ordination ceremony, she requested that the laying on of hands be done by her Medical Mission sisters. Betsy believes that she was the first person in the last century to be ordained by a Lutheran and Episcopal bishop at the same time.

At each step, Betsy's journey fortified her understanding of loss and the adaptation to loss, even when the losses were ultimate in her life. She saw her holy work as an extension of God's desire that we not only make the most out of life but that we hear the unfiltered lessons that death teaches and grow from them. We shouldn't leave unfinished emotional business for another generation to sort through without answers. We only have now.

Betsy's e-mail address begins with the words "Old Bat." She has a healthy disregard for aging and a sense of humor that has carried her through some very dark hours. I mentioned a friend who was struggling with the fact that her mother had just started hospice care. She was in denial that death was around the corner. I was worried about her. Betsy put her arm around me and said, "Tell her to give me a call. I'd love to speak to her." And I knew that she meant it.

I've been thinking about Betsy for months, especially when putting off visiting someone who is sick because I'm worried about myself. There's no better way to say it. I know that every time I go to a hospital I'm facing my own mortality. And I don't want to. I'm not comfortable there. I hate the disinfectant smell that only thinly masks the smell of sickness and death. I want to make a quick visit, fulfill my obligation, pay my parking ticket and race out of there. In my heart, I know that being there for people who are sick and dying is the right thing to do, especially when they have unfinished business. Betsy forced me into a certain kind of honesty when it comes to that fear. She made me think about all the conversations we're *not* having with people we love who are aging or very sick. We don't discuss their fears or their longings or what they would like to see happen in the time they have left. We clutter conversations with momentary concerns but not the deeper emotional issues of a lifetime. Why aren't we having them?

It's hard to talk about dying because we don't always have the language or someone like Betsy in our lives to coax it out of us. When Betsy ran support groups for the dying, she learned to help people express and face their deepest fears about dying, and she began to understand that not everyone has the language or the emotional strength to talk about her own death or the death of the one she loves. Kübler-Ross in her book on life after death believes that the soul knows when it is approaching death and needs a way to express this time and its challenges:

> The truth is the patient knows he or she is dying through the natural knowledge of the soul. Not to speak about this process is to deny the human being the essential need to complete unfinished business by collecting the fragments of the soul that long to come together before the soul is called home. It is that completion that ultimately brings the soul peace and calm, making it ready to release itself from this earthly life. And completion requires open dialogue with friends, family members, business associates, and even adversaries.[6]

Betsy intuitively understands this need and also understands that most dying people and their families do not know how to go about completing unfinished emotional business. So she made it her business. Initially she wasn't sure what to do; it was an evolving process. "But I learned that there was a good way to die and a *not* good way to die. I wanted to make the end a positive time."

Betsy's energy comes out in her hands and her voice. Even seated in her study with her two small dogs jumping on and off her lap, she seemed alive with a sense of purpose. Her yard was filled with hyacinths and daffodils that had just begun to bloom. Joy and peace surrounded her. This was especially evident later when her grandson and granddaughter burst in and, like the dogs, jumped all over her. She greeted them with loving enthusiasm, and I could only imagine what consolation it would be to be under Betsy's care if my own life were coming to an end. Betsy has another remarkable gift. She speaks with an easy self-confidence and self-knowledge about very painful subjects. She offers this ease to her patients because she knows that the inability to talk about death often leads to the indignity of dying.

Dr. Ira Byock, the former president of the American Academy of Hospice and Palliative Medicine and author of *Dying Well*, contrasts the unfinished business of an abrupt death with the kind of slow and incremental death that should allow the dying to take care of their emotional odds and ends, which "includes the chance to reconcile strained relationships, perhaps between previous spouses, or between a parent and an estranged adult child. . . . Even at the very end of life, healing a relationship can transform the history of a family. A relationship that is complete need not end; in this context, complete means there is nothing left unsaid or undone.[7] Byock opens his book with a detailed discussion of his own father's death, a man who died in his home under his care and the care of his family. He observed: "Dad's dying was certainly not the happiest time in our family's life, but as a family we had never been more intimate, more open, or more openly loving. His death allowed us, I could say, forced us, to talk about the things that mattered . . . family, our relationships with each other, our shared past, and the unknown future. We reminisced about good times and bad."[8]

Betsy's intuitive way of handling unfinished business gained support from a well-known piece of research published in 1989 in *Lancet*, a prestigious medical journal.[9] Dr. David Spiegel from Stanford University conducted years of research to prove that women with metastasized breast cancer could live longer if they had what he calls supportive-expressive group therapy. Control and variable groups of women with almost no chance of recovery were studied to determine if participation once a week in a support group was beneficial. Spiegel discovered that the control subjects lived an average of 18.9 months, while those receiving group therapy lived 36.6 months. Talking with others about fears that could not be easily shared with family and friends actually extended life.

This research generated great optimism in the handling of a brutal disease and spawned support groups not only for women with metastasized breast cancer but also for people with other fatal diseases. People found that being able to speak openly about illness and death comforted them, relieved them of the loneliness of cancer, and helped them speak with family members and friends about what was happening to them. Many women wanted to speak frankly about cancer, but their families were not ready or able to be that honest. Though a 2004 study questioned Spiegel's research,[10] support group participation does have many other benefits, including helping people cope with a diagnosis, even if it does not help survival rates. Group discussions help men and women find a voice where they may feel silenced among peers and loved ones. They can enhance life's quality at the end if not its duration.

Communication with the dying can be halting and difficult. Well-meaning people try to smooth things over or minimize an illness by proclaiming the patient's good luck that it's not something else or something worse: "Well, at least you've got a good cancer."

In the words of one nurse who works with the dying, such talk can cheapen the experience and make the ending of a life more unbearable.

Burying our thoughts and feelings can seem like protection, but it actually leads to isolation, for both caregivers and patients. Silence begets silence, loneliness, or depression. The person thinks: *This is too hard for the people around me. I'd better take care of their fears and discomforts instead of my own.* So the sick person takes over the role of caregiver, avoids talking about anything that will upset the family, and in so doing further isolates him- or herself. Meanwhile the caregiver thinks: *If I acknowledge what's happening, it will be too overwhelming to handle.*[11]

David Kessler, a leader in the field of hospice and palliative care and author of *The Needs of the Dying*, advises that people not have difficult conversations about death outside the hospital room or bedroom where the dying cannot participate in a discussion of their own last days. When it comes to the dying, we make decisions unknown to them, talk about them without them in the room or act as if they have already died when they are not yet taken from us. In acting this way, we fail to honor them and their last wishes.[12]

This reminds me of a joke. Bernie was on his deathbed when he smelled the wonderful combination of cinnamon and yeast wafting its way upstairs to his bedroom. Bernie called for his daughter and in a plaintive voice said, "Ethel, give a dying man his last wish. Bring me a piece of your mother's delicious babka." Ethel went downstairs but came back up empty-handed. "Sorry, Pa. Mom says it's for after."

Kessler, a close friend of Elisabeth Kübler-Ross and who was present when she died, writes that although these talks are challenging, they must be had, precisely because these words stay embedded deeply in our memories:

At times you may feel as if you're walking on eggshells, but everyone should be allowed to say what needs to be said. This is a sacred time because of the authenticity of the emotions that occur. We must let ourselves and our loved ones express feelings and emotions, no matter what the reactions may be. . . . These feelings are among the purest found in life. Honoring these expressions is a holy obligation we have to each other.[13]

Kessler met Mother Teresa before she passed away and told her about his book. He asked her what he should tell people about death. She replied, "Tell them not to be afraid of dying. It is very simple. The dying need tender loving, nothing more."

I myself had the privilege to visit a Mother Teresa clinic for the dying in Addis Ababa, Ethiopia, in 2006. What I witnessed shook up any notion I had of a shadowy space filled with the sighs of the near dead. The facility has large connecting rooms where every space is taken up by rows of beds covered in colorful blankets. In virtually each bed, someone is dying. Yet there was nothing depressing about it. People walked into the facility to die because they did not want to die alone. Very few patients in this clinic had any chance of recovery. But that did not stop some remarkable doctors and nurses from easing their suffering at the end. I met a woman whose cheek was totally disfigured by a growth that had blown up the entire right side of her face. She was smiling and speaking as if it were just another ordinary day. And I saw, as I walked among the beds speaking with people like her, that there was tremendous peacefulness in the room, a transcendent sort of quiet punctuated by laughter and also by howls of pain. It was a room full of dignity. The clinic is not there to offer them false hope. It offers them community. It gives them basic human respect. It is a place that offers sanctity of the body and preparation for the soul for its last moments on earth.

• • •

Women and men like Betsy dedicate their careers to not letting the dying exit life anonymously. They devote themselves to witnessing death and helping people identify what is holding them back from full acceptance of death and then getting them to the point of acceptance, both for those who are dying and their caregivers. Most often the obstacle is something left unsaid or undone. David Kuhl, a physician and expert in palliative care, observes that not removing the barriers to unfinished business generates more suffering:

> It takes physical, psychic and spiritual energy to suffer. When a person's energy must go toward coping with pain, nausea, vomiting, restlessness, insomnia, anxiety, or depression, he or she is not free to focus on anything else, especially on taking care of unfinished business and writing the last chapter of his or her life in a way that is a fitting tribute to that life.[14]

If someone else can help the person who is dying refocus on unfinished business, then death can feel less frightening and even, as Betsy observed, welcome. Betsy sees this work as her personal mission.

"I once had a patient," Betsy said, "who gave birth to a daughter in India and, at one stage, was given medicine that was later associated with cervical cancer in daughters." The woman was very anxious about this secret she had been holding on to for decades. Suddenly, she felt she had to know if the medicine she was given was indeed this one, so that she could warn her daughter. She didn't want her daughter to go through the same hell she faced. "She didn't remember the names of her doctors all those years ago, but she did remember that she was in a Holy Family hospital in India. I got in contact with the hospital since it was associated with my nursing order, and it turns out her ob-gyn was a sister I actually knew from my own training. They told me that they never used that kind of medicine in Holy Family hospitals." The woman was immensely relieved. Betsy was able to reassure her patient that this secret and its potential consequences would not follow her to the grave. It helped her patient let go. It prepared her to accept death.

I often hear people mention the unfinished business of life in the same breath as the idea of granting permission for a person to die. Sometimes not having taken care of a problem, particularly one of an emotional nature, holds people back from dying. Alternatively, people who believe they are needed or depended upon for one reason or another often hold on until they are told by those who they perceive are dependent on them that they are free to go. "I wonder if they told him that he has permission to die," a friend wondered when a relative's elderly and frail father was hanging on to a very tenuous life. "I remember with my grandmother," she remarked, "that we were told to go into her room and tell her we love her and say goodbye and let her know that she has our permission to die." She died only hours later. Whether or not there was a correlation remains a mystery, but it seemed to the family that this was critical to her release.

Because there is so much anxiety around these awkward conversations and requests, the hospice movement provides critical aid in helping families create a loving, warm passage to death. Yet statistically, only a third of terminally ill patients in the United States take advantage of hospice care, even though hospices, or at least the idea of them, have been around since the early medieval period. The word *hospice* is derived from the Latin *hospes*, which refers to both guests and hosts. At its root, hospice was a network of institutions offering hospitality rather than help coping with illness. Convents and monasteries as early as the eleventh century used to open their doors to tired and ailing travelers, ensuring that they would receive the proper food and housing they required. Over time, church refuges were created for the very ill who may have felt lost, helpless or companionless at their time of greatest vulnerability. Taking care of the sickest in society was regarded as an act of bottomless compassion and mercy. By the fourteenth century, the first official hospice, the Knights Hospitaller of St. John of Jerusalem, was opened in Rhodes. France opened a number of such refuges in the seventeenth century, but it was not until the nineteenth century that the idea of a special care facility for the dying received international attention. A clinic in London, the Friedenheim, opened in 1892 to care for patients dying of tuberculosis. It had only thirty-five beds. In the decades that followed more such facilities were created in Great Britain and elsewhere in the British Commonwealth. America followed suit, and in 1899 St. Rose's Hospice by the Servants for Relief of Incurable Cancer opened in New York and spread to six other locations around the country.

One of the pioneers of the modern hospice movement was Dame Cicely Saunders, who died in 2005. Like Betsy, Cicely was a registered nurse who worked closely with terminally ill patients and understood the importance of helping them and their families deal with pain management and the psychological and spiritual challenges that accompany the last few months of life. Cicely actually fell in love with a dying patient, David Tasma, a Jewish-Polish refugee from the Warsaw ghetto. He left her £500 after he died so that she could live comfortably as a "window" [sic]. After Tasma died, Cicely began to work on a volunteer basis at St. Luke's Home for the Dying Poor in London. A doctor advised her that the best way to change medical policy was to become a doctor herself, so Cicely bravely went to medical school in the 1950s, at a time when few women pursued MDs as a profession. She took her qualifying exams in 1957 and passed.

Cicely started her own facility, St. Christopher's Hospice, in the late 1960s after being inspired by a verse in Psalm 37: "Commit thy way unto the Lord; trust also in Him; and He shall bring it to pass." She had a symbolic pane of glass installed in the building to honor Tasma's last wish that she be a window, making a spelling error into a symbolic statement of hope. On a tour of America to spread the gospel of better deaths for the terminally ill, Cicely got the attention of a dean at the Yale nursing school who heard her speak. This dean then spent a month under Cicely's mentorship in London and brought her ideas back to the United States in the form of Hospice Inc., a movement that began in the United States in the early 1970s. Cicely earned accolades and some of the most prestigious honors given in Britain. She died of cancer in 2005 in the very facility she created. In her own words, her philosophy of death was simple: "You matter because you are you, and you matter to the end of your life. We will do all we can not only to help you die peacefully, but also to live until you die." This expression "to live until you die" underlies the work that hospices do and that people like Betsy do. They know that life is ending but also that it has not ended.

Hospice is not a religious movement (although hospice workers will provide clergy assistance to the dying and their caregivers if requested). It is a movement to ease the end of life for the dying and their caregivers, usually in their own homes but sometimes in designated facilities. Dr. Ira Byock writes how distressing it is when people fight to the death instead of accepting death and enjoying the last days, weeks or months of life. He dislikes the term "the good death," since it fails to capture the complexity of the human condition. In Byock's words: "Good death connotes a formulaic or prescriptive approach to life's end, as if a good outcome chiefly depended on the right mix of people, place, medications, and services."[15]

Byock prefers the phrase "dying well" because for him it refers to a sense of living *and* a process of dying. He finds that this is what hospice care provides for the terminally ill: the chance to die well. In particular, Byock singles out the challenges of death in the hospital when hospitalization could have been avoided and the patient could have died more peacefully at home, without the glare of ambulance lights, the noise of sirens and the pain that transport alone can inflict. Nursing homes routinely send patients close to death to the hospital so that they can claim lower mortality rates without concern for the dignity of the closing moments of a life. Byock recommends hospice care as a way to introduce patients and their families to death slowly and gently, letting the last slice of life be celebrated. Like Betsy, he believes the last weeks of a person's life can be an inspiring and precious time to take care of unfinished concerns and anxieties and express love.

It can also become a time of spiritual awakening. It reinforces something that we know latently but rarely confront: we are not in ultimate control of our lives. G. Leigh Wilkerson, a registered nurse, has written several pamphlets that many hospice workers give out routinely. Wilkerson, like so many hospice nurses and medical workers, recognizes the defensiveness, anger and shame associated with the weeks leading up to death. Her guide *Considering Comfort Care* helps families think about transitioning a family member or friend into hospice care, understanding that the decision to enter hospice is often the hardest part.[16] Wilkerson got involved in the hospice movement because, like Betsy, she too saw the problem of hospital deaths and the ignominy of the dying in strictly medical settings:

> When I was a nurse, I saw many people spend the last days of their lives surrounded by machines, alarms and busy staff. It was not a place where loved ones could sit and hold a hand, or tell family stories. There was no preparation for loss; no time for heartfelt words. The hospital staff was focused on saving lives (as we want them to

be in a critical-care unit) and unable to help families prepare for the end of life. I saw people pass away without ever being able to say the goodbyes we would all want them to say.[17]

Wilkerson's experience as a hospice nurse helped her see a more natural and compassionate way of dying. Research on hospice care tells us that patients actually live longer when they are in a nurturing home environment.[18] Hospice care is not only available for cancer patients but anyone facing the last months of their lives with a terminal illness. Hospice recommends a six-month window to transition the dying gradually into the embrace of death and help the family prepare emotionally and spiritually.

It takes a person with Wilkerson's experience to stress that comfort care is not giving up hope, stopping everything, quitting, losing the battle, just letting someone die or doing nothing. Hospice emphasizes that the comfort care process is not a statement of resignation but a change of heart in the perception and recognition that death is approaching and that there comes a time to begin the separation process and say goodbye and do so with the minimum amount of pain and the maximum amount of love. Wilkerson emphasizes that you can stop hospice care at any time if you're getting better.

Wilkerson warns that sometimes the hospice approach can be sabotaged by a late-visiting relative or friend who is shocked that the family is "giving up" because they are allowing a hospice team to take over the patient's care. This sudden outcry can undo months of painful preparation in a single blow, harping on heartstrings and surfacing guilt.

Hospice professionals and volunteers often ask the caregivers and family to slow down and match the pace of the dying. Don't rush stories. Take time to listen and hold hands. The last and best gift you can give the dying may be relieving the worries of a loved one by being a patient listener and not a dominating talker.

People who are dying often need really good pain management as well, and this is where hospice is again a godsend. Betsy recalled that in her early nursing years dying patients were practically ignored. She recalls seeing the terminally ill shunted as far as possible from the nursing station. If they were dying, they did not exist. They were an inconvenience to the profession. "But dying people are still living," Betsy said. "And I can do something about the quality of that living." She even tried to get heroin legalized for those who were dying and in need of extreme pain management but was unsuccessful.

Hospice volunteers often have to manage certain unarticulated assumptions people have about pain. Pain is not inevitable. It is not an expected part of death that people have to suffer with or through. Some people believe that pain is a spiritual punishment and that it builds character and offers redemption. The act of suffering in this world exempts one from suffering in the next world. Many ancient religions depict illness in this very way, leading some to negate the role of physicians, healers and traditional medicine. If God made a person sick there must be a reason, and it is not for us to interfere with the divine plan. Some believe, even without a pronounced or acknowledged spiritual tradition, that pain is natural. Most experts on the experience of dying take the opposite view and suggest that denying palliative or comfort care is one of the worst ways to manage end-of-life issues. If you can ameliorate your own pain or the pain of others, and you don't use your resources to manage your emotional landscape, then you deny yourself and your caregivers a better death.

Gingerly, I took a step in Betsy's direction. I am very close with my ninety-nine-year-old grandmother. We call her "Bubbie," the Yiddish word for "grandmother"; mostly, I call her "Bubs," with an occasional "Bubbilicious."

My grandparents were married for seventy-two years when Zeide passed away. Bubs lives with me for the summers to escape the humidity of Florida. We speak every night on the phone in the winter. She gives me a daily weather report and discusses her dinner.

Bubbie is of the old school Jewish extraction, and superstition courses through her blood. I knew that having a talk with her about unfinished business was not going to be easy. For her, most unfinished business is not going to be resolved, because she can never bring back her parents and her siblings who were killed, or undo the anguish of her past. It all gets lost in the large, unanswerable questions of how humans could be so cruel and how God could be so absent. When she talks about it she balls her fists, and you can see the anger. It's palpable even all these years later.

She's done much in her life and is ready to go. But the problem is that she's in perfectly good health. Nevertheless, if you ask her anything about the immediate future, she is always pessimistic:

"How many days left do I have, really?"

"I can't make any plans. I could go any minute."

"I need this sweater like a hole in the head. No, I need a hole in the head more. Who's going to see me wear it? No one cares from an old lady."

"You should live and be well. Me? I'm finished."

She talks about dying all the time, so how hard could it be to have a real talk with her about death? Betsy inspired me to try a difficult conversation with her about her own death. No more jokes and innuendos. No more superstitions. A real conversation. I wanted to know if she had regrets or if there was someone she wanted to talk to about the past. Perhaps there was someone she needed to ask forgiveness from. Maybe there was something she needed but was afraid to ask. We sat on the front porch of my house, in her favorite spot, in the late afternoon when the sun warms the flagstones.

"So, Bubs, I wanted to talk to you about something. Is now a good time?"

"Do I have something else to do?"

"Well, now that you're getting older, I thought maybe we could talk about your dying. I mean, not that we want you to go, God forbid. I just thought that maybe there's something that you still want to do before you die. Maybe we could make it happen."

It was deadly silent for a few minutes. I watched the dust motes swirl in the sunshine and waited for an answer.

"You trying to kill me?"

## Chapter Seven

# Closing Words

Bob was so shy in high school that he couldn't bring himself to ask Sally out despite his huge crush on her. One day his best friend, George, locked him in the basement and wouldn't let him out until he asked Sally on a date. That was the start of a long life together for Bob and Sally. When Bob's granddaughter asked him for advice about marriage before her own wedding, Bob claimed he was no expert but said, "You see Sally and me as old folks, but I can tell you, to me, Sally is more beautiful than when we married because I've learned who she really is—what a wonderful person she is." Bob described Sally as a mysterious lover who became a loyal roommate. "I'm with her from morning to night and love it." Two days short of their sixty-seventh anniversary, she died. Bob's last words to Sally were "You made my life."[1]

Contrast this with the hotel emperor Conrad Hilton's apocryphal last words when he died in 1979: "Leave the shower curtain on the inside of the tub." Karl Marx had no patience for a meaningful exclamation mark with his last breath: "Go on, get out! Last words are for fools who haven't said enough." So much for Marx. Then again, look at the state of communism today.

The words we leave behind really *do* matter. The very last words sometimes matter the most. Knowing this, we want the dying and the living to craft last words that create positive associations with the moment of death and its aftermath.

Some people text each other or write notes so that there is some kind of printed word that makes a lasting impression when time is urgently leaving us. Survivors still speak of phone messages they received from friends and loved ones who did not make it on 9/11. Moises Rivas, who worked in the North Tower, left his wife, Elizabeth, one last present. He managed to get through by phone to his stepdaughter and leave a message for her to pass on to his wife: "He loves you no matter what. He loves you." Mark Bingham called his mother to say goodbye from United Airlines Flight 93. His mother, Alice Hoglan, holds on to those words. "He said, 'I want you to know I love you very much, and I'm calling you from the plane. We've been taken over. There are three men who say they've got a bomb.'"

Melissa Harrington, a young international trade consultant at the World Trade Center, was able to get through to her father, who tried, in a calm, assuring manner, to get her to the stairwell and out of the building. As the smoke grew thicker, they told each other that they loved each other and then Melissa had a message to pass on to her newlywed husband, whom she could not reach. "You have to do me a favor. You have to call Sean and tell him where I am and tell him that I love him." Twelve minutes later, Melissa managed to leave her own message for her husband: "Sean, it's me. I just wanted to let you know I love you, and I'm stuck in this building in New York. There's a lot of smoke, and I just wanted to let you know that I love you always." And those were Melissa's last recorded words.

You will often hear someone at a funeral share last words or last messages, like a full stop at the end of a sentence, a small act of punctuation. Tragically, suicide notes, awful as they are, serve this function: to explain or to say goodbye. These are usually one-sided partings that leave no opportunity for the living to respond, as we might do with an ordinary letter. But worse are those who leave this world without final words, leaving family and friends dazed, confused and guilty. In the place where words should explain is a towering emptiness, a black hole of uncertainty.

To prevent this, a friend and rabbinic colleague of mine made one of his boldest sermons a public closure of sorts. Jack got up in front of his congregation on Yom Kippur and talked about his death. He looked at and spoke directly to his family, who were seated eight rows back from the pulpit. His message was blunt and open. I heard about it from him, but, more importantly: I heard about it first from a congregant in the audience two days after the holiday. I saw my friend Julie in a school parking lot in Virginia. I casually asked her how her holidays were and got a response I don't often hear: "They were amazing. My rabbi gave a sermon that I just can't shake." She told me all about it and then I asked Jack myself for a copy.

He told his congregation that he was perfectly healthy but that he had an important issue to discuss: his dying. His father had died at sixty-five. He was fifty-nine. He gauged the emotional temperature of a congregation he had shepherded for twenty-five years: "We are all going to cry, especially the members of my family who already know what is in this sermon. But if I can do this in front of all of you, emotional coward that I mostly am, then you can do this privately with the people you love. And you must."

Jack spoke about his love for his family and his pride in each of them. He told them that when he ages, he does not mind becoming somewhat of a burden on his family, since "each of you has been a burden I have carried at some point in my life, and they were the happiest burdens I can remember." But he didn't want to be afflicted with an illness so badly that its lasting memory would leave the permanent image of a decimated self with them. He told them that when his body surrendered itself that he would look back on his life with gratitude: "If I have to look back at what I have accomplished in this world I only have to look at you and know that I am leaving the world a better place than I found it." Jack wanted his family to be sure of all these feelings and to leave none of them unspoken. He asked forgiveness of his congregation for opening his life to them with a "Talmudic style scrutiny" and for any upset that he caused them. He told them how much he loved them as well, leaving no feeling to chance. He left last words to help them leave last words.

Few people confront death like this because word preparation is a choice that few people make; usually it is only those with an intimate and constant dread of death, those facing terminal illness or those in dangerous, life-threatening jobs. Many soldiers, for example, write living wills or ethical wills or letters to those they love with a final goodbye, "in the event that . . ." A soldier overseas who was going into a very difficult skirmish in the Middle East actually left a letter and vials of sperm for his fiancée in the event that he never made it back alive. He didn't, and while the children born from this vial can never compensate for the loss, his parents have grandchildren who are a beautiful extension of a son who never lived to see them.

When people are dying of illness, writer Marianne Williamson in her book A Return to Love recommends that they write a letter to their illness that allows them to personify and express their full anger at its pillaging of the body.[2] This personification and communication strangely offer people a little more control over what is happening to them. Not only do they have last words for those they love, sick people should have last words about their condition, and to the very sickness that placed them in the position in the first place. Through the process, people come to uncover secret fears and expectations, dashed hopes and unexpected courage.

Last words take another format: obituaries, the words that someone else uses to describe your life once it's over. You can't really be immortalized in the newspaper because nothing seems more impermanent than yesterday's news or yesterday's deaths. I scan the paper and what immediately strikes me is the hierarchy of the obituary page. The "Pioneering French Egyptologist" got a photo and three columns of text. She wrote dozens of books, two of which were bestsellers in France, and she was not even a citizen of this country. A local teacher, a lawyer and a conference coordinator each got a five-paragraph tribute, as did a food service worker at a local university who coached youth baseball for two decades. And then there were the paid ads, the death notices, which only got a paragraph of condensed text. Some had a photo. Some did not. Depends what you paid for.

Finding the right words to memorialize the dead has a history all its own. Obituaries as a standard feature in newspapers probably emerged incrementally in American newspapers from the 1870s to 1900. There were death notices as early as the 1830s but not as a regular segment of the newspaper. National papers cover people of national significance. Local papers cover local deaths. But significance is relative, as anyone knows who feels that his or her deceased has been slighted by an omission.

Some people read obits every day; some people even clip out inspiring or odd obits and file them. Others find that as they age they begin to turn to these pages to look for friends and the celebrities of their era. Marilyn Johnson went from reading obits obsessively to writing them and then writing a whole book about writing them, *The Dead Beat: Lost Souls, Lucky Stiffs, and the Perverse Pleasures of Obituaries*. Johnson calls it the art of writing history "as it is happening." She claims that once you start reading, obits can provoke addictions and "can take you to the heroin level in no time."[3]

How does a perfectly nice journalist end up writing obituaries? Most start out writing obits on the bottom of the newspaper chain and work their way up to the living. Some love the genre and stay. Many obit writers have nicknames, like Doyenne of Death, Dr. Death, Angel of Death, and Black Mariah. (The last is the name of the paddy wagon used to transport those who just died. Drivers often robbed the corpses before burial.) According to Johnson, most long-term obit writers are experienced journalists, usually in their fifties, who were once English majors. She describes herself as a socially unfit lover of the genre: "This tight little coil of biography with its literary flourishes reminds us of a poem. Certainly it contains the most creative writing in journalism."[4] The world is littered with unemployed but wonderfully employable English majors who might just take up the field if backed by the right skill set. Johnson does not disappoint. She tells us exactly what she thinks you need to be a good obituary writer: reporting skills and life experience. A good sense of humor is helpful, as is empathy, but neither is essential. Then there is the intangible skill, something Johnson has trouble pinning down: "an ability to weigh someone's life and accomplishments historically, in the context of the times. A good obit writer has to communicate the significance of a person, a place, an era . . . to capture a person with economy and grace, and work in the hurricane of emotion that swirls around the newly dead."[5]

Writing about the dead is a skill, maybe even an art form, and avoiding clichés about death requires craftsmanship. That's why the

SPOW awards are important; they raise the literary standard. The Society of Professional Obituary Writers convenes annually to discuss terrific obits, changing styles and the challenges of writing about people who can't write a letter to the editor if they hate what you wrote. The obit writer is a person of mystery to newspaper readers, which is only enhanced by the words used to describe one well-known obit writer's boss: "God is my assignment editor." By virtue of their jobs, obit writers seem to know more about the ends and beginnings of most of the people who matter. Amelia Rosner, another obit writer, sums it up rather neatly: "We know who's sick and who's dying, and we know how many of the original cast members of *Gilligan's Island* are still alive."

In 2008, Jim Nicholson of the *Philadelphia Daily News* became the first recipient of the SPOW lifetime achievement award. Nicholson, a pioneer in writing obits about ordinary people, once said, "A little life well lived is worth telling about." Where the obit writer typically covers the famous and people of personal or professional renown, Nicholson focuses on telling the story of the common folk, the small and mundane details that constitute a life. Nicholson redefined the terms of significance in his genre.

Nicholson was touched by the award: "Love the tombstone shape."[6] Kay Powell, who writes obits for the *Atlanta Journal-Constitution*, won the SPOW, also known as the Grimmy Award, for the best body of work in 2007 and shared it in 2008. Her two awards sit side by side in her office, reminding her of the Ten Commandments. You can also win an award for the best obit about a celebrity, the best long obit and the best obit about your average Joe.

You've got to be good at your job if you want to profile really famous dead people. Johnson has written obits for Princess Di, Jackie Onassis, Katharine Hepburn, Johnny Cash, Bob Hope and Marlon Brando. In Johnson's field, name-dropping takes on a whole new meaning. The first famous person obit Johnson ever snagged was

Rock Hudson, which, not coincidentally, was the first time his story, particularly his offscreen life as a homosexual, was told publicly. This obituary was actually more than news. It was a scoop!

There is a template that most obit writers follow. The first sentence of an obit offers the reader a wealth of information and generally contains a clause or a phrase offset by commas that generally appears right after the name. It has been called "the who clause," "the comma" or "the descriptive." British obituaries, according to Johnson, are generally lower key in the descriptive, not offering the cause of death right away and not belaboring the medical details of death that often feature in American obits. The British prefer their descriptives lean, with only the date and location of death. Later follows "the bad news" or "death sentence," the paragraph or paragraphs that detail what actually happened as far as the loss of life is concerned. Then there is "the song and dance" or "the tombstone," the information that communicates the sparkle or dazzle of the deceased's life. This is usually followed by what some obit writers call "the desperate chronology," namely what the deceased did over the course of a life, the details of normal life: birth, marriage, positions held, children. Johnson adds the term "colorful quotes" to describe what friends, colleagues, relatives or fans have to say about the person. These quotes add personality to the life being described. Johnson offers this parable to help us understand the significance of the quote in the obit: "Imagine a round table, and the people who knew the deceased standing up, rapping on their glasses with a spoon, and saying something that fills in the blanks, directly or indirectly."[7] This might be followed by a punchline of some sort, a zinger that adds spice to the chronology. Finally, the typical obit ends with a "list of survivors," which is hard to capture creatively, although some obit writers tuck it in earlier so that they can end their columns with more sizzle.

To nab this lingo and range well, obit writers make sure that celebrities and politicians have their obituaries written well in advance of their deaths and keep them updated regularly to be sure that when the moment comes, the piece is ready for press. You've really made it if you have your own obituary years before you actually die. On the status front, it beats a chauffeur and a vacation home in Nantucket any day.

Kate Zernike co-authored the *New York Times* obit for Osama bin Laden on a tight deadline in 2001, but her 4,000 words waited another ten years for a public appearance. By the time the obit appeared in 2011, her co-author had already died. The *Columbia Journalism Review* interviewed Zernike about her thoughts on bin Laden's death in the intervening ten years. A long obit is called a "double truck" in obit insider jargon, and that's what the *Times* felt that bin Laden deserved: two full pages on this king of terrorism. As Zernike waited and waited for the news, she thought that bin Laden's profile in the world was diminishing and that the *Times* would never run the full two pages, maybe just one. When the news finally broke, papers the world over scrambled to see what they had on file. The *Times* pulled up and published the old obit with few additions and without informing Zernike. Zernike wondered if the obit would withstand the test of time, but as she read it at a distance, she realized that it had.

The *Journalism Review* asked if Zernike believed that bin Laden deserved an obituary. She answered cautiously: "I think a lot of people read obituaries to learn something about life, about how the world works, and about what individual stories tell us about some universal idea." Given that bin Laden was such a significant figure in modern world history, it seemed only right to have an obituary.

We all probably wonder if we'll ever make it into the *Times* or the local rag in the end. I confess: I secretly hope for a double truck. I feel a lot of pressure.

Some people will do odd things to get attention, even once they're already dead. There are pranksters and hoaxers who submit obituaries for people who have not died, either out of revenge or just to get a laugh. Probably the most famous in this category was staged by the jazz musician and mockumentarist Alan Abel. Near a ski lodge in 1979, Abel pretended he had a heart attack, and a fake funeral director picked up his things. A team of twelve people were involved in the attention-getting hoax. A woman who pretended to be his wife gave notice to the *New York Times*; the paper printed his obituary in early January of that year:

> Alan Abel, a writer, musician and film producer who specialized in satire and lampoons, died of a heart attack yesterday at Sundance, a ski resort near Orem, Utah, while investigating a location for a new film. He was 50 years old and lived in Manhattan and Westport, Conn.
>
> Mr. Abel, a graduate of Ohio State University with majors in music and speech, made a point in his work of challenging the obvious and uttering the outrageous. He gained national recognition several years ago when he mounted a campaign for animal decency, demanding that horses and dogs, for example, be fitted with underwear.

On January 3, the day after the obituary appeared, Abel went from staging his funeral to staging a press conference, where he announced that he was still alive, borrowing Mark Twain's famous words: "Reports of my demise have been grossly exaggerated." The editor of the *Times* was furious and vowed never to have Abel's name in print in his paper again. Abel was a PR master, however, and the editor was unable to keep his vow. Not long after his resurrection, Abel wrote about a school for panhandlers—a total fiction, naturally—and was the mastermind behind seven people fainting on the set of the *Phil Donahue Show*. The man was unstoppable.

While Mr. Abel did not seem to take the task of last words seriously, many others do. In late medieval Europe, a time and place beset by disease and plagues, people actually rehearsed their funerals. Death was a likely visitor in most homes, so the thinking was "practice makes perfect." Believing that this would help people confront the reality of illness, people used a guidebook. Two Latin texts became popular with medieval Christians, both called *Ars bene moriendi*, or "The Art of Dying Well." There was a longer and shorter text, often accompanied by woodcut illustrations (usually disturbingly graphic), which were especially helpful for the illiterate who could understand the pictures even if the words eluded them. Those who could read popularized these guides, and for the next centuries they traveled across Europe, translated into multiple languages.

Death was not something to fear, according to the *Ars bene moriendi*, but there are sins that dying people should avoid, like impatience, despair and lack of faith. Death presents ample opportunities for repentance, which these guides heartily recommend, and the books contain prayers for the dying to achieve atonement and leave the world with sanctified words. Friends and relatives are also offered recommendations on how to behave toward the dying and the correct spiritual posture to assume at this time.

Today at a kibbutz in the north of Israel, Beit Hashita, known for its famous canned garlic-flavored pickles, you can't quite rehearse your death but you can be in charge of your last words through your memory drawer. The kibbutz was founded in 1928, twenty years before the establishment of the state. For years it had seen too many wars and was struggling to find a way to memorialize eleven soldiers killed in the Yom Kippur War. A composer decided to set a prayer from the Yom Kippur service to a haunting melody and have a concert on Yom Kippur. The kibbutz members were largely secular, and it seemed somewhat strange to pick a solemn petition for compassion from a traditional prayerbook. Nevertheless, the kibbutz continues to hold a concert every year, and the haunting melody has traveled into many traditional services, seizing on the existential language of the prayer," "who will die a timely death and who an untimely death," to capture the universal sentiment of fear and loss.

But the kibbutz did more than memorialize the dead. This event inspired the kibbutz membership to give more thought to last words. They created a "Memorial Room" at the center of the kibbutz; in the shadow of the eleven deaths, the kibbutz decided to help its extended family preserve their personal memories for those after them. Each member of the kibbutz is allotted a drawer in the Memorial Room to preserve important documents and memories that he or she would like to archive for future generations. The death drawer is your own. You pick what you would like to put inside.

Sometimes when we don't have last words, we have last things. Remember Rose? She made sure that Connie and her sisters took what they wanted during her lifetime to avoid strife afterward. Writer Jo Myers offers guidance on last things in her guide to preparing for the end of life, *Good to Go*. One of the best lines in the book is an endorsement by a comedian on the first page: "If you or someone you know will die someday, read Jo's book." (Myers subtitles her chapter on cremation "Making an Ash of Yourself"). Myers writes that there always seems to be some "seemingly innocuous item" that can cause a rift among survivors. Usually the problem is not the item itself. "It might represent deeper, unexplored matters of which neither party is aware."[8] Presenting items to a loved one can be an act of great importance and intimacy that speaks to the relationship between giver and receiver. A will never communicates the transaction of love the way that giving the item does in your lifetime. Not only can you not take it with you; you aren't going to enjoy it until the very last day. Isn't it better knowing where an item will go and who will be entrusted with its care while you are still alive? As people age, they often make a habit of giving items away on special occasions. Myers also advises making a home movie of the parent or friend bequeathing items because it is much more personal than a lawyer reading a document. Myers probably never realized that she was advising a very ancient biblical practice. The Bible says that right before he died, "Abraham gave gifts while he was still living."[9]

My friend Sarah has an unusual gift from her grandfather that has no monetary worth whatsoever. She keeps it in her office and is often answering the question "What's that?" to visitors. Her grandfather retired from public service and lived on a boat for over twenty years. His passion was being on the water, and he loved everything nautical. He was content to be the captain of his boat and sail it up and down the East Coast. When he died, the family went through his things and divided them up. Sarah noticed that many of her grandfather's possessions had made it into her father's study. Her father kept two paperweights on his desk that her grandfather used in order to hold down his maps when he was going to chart the course for his next trip. "When my twin sister and I turned twenty-five, my father said a bunch of times, 'I don't know what to get you.' He always tries to give us something meaningful. Then he called and said, 'I've found the perfect thing.'" Turning twenty-five is a big milestone, and Sarah's dad always includes long and beautiful cards with his birthday gifts, telling his girls how proud he is and blessing them with hopes for the coming year. "I opened the package and it took me a few minutes to register what it was and then I said, 'I know what this is.' And it was such an incredible gift." There it was: a narrow, flat, metal-gray lead weight with a rounded point on one side. You could walk by it in your backyard and not notice it. But for Sarah, this weight has special significance. "My dad wrote that his father used it to chart his course and that we should think of him as we chart ours. Like my grandfather, I also went into nonprofit work, and when I look at the weight on my desk, I feel like I am carrying on his legacy. I feel connected to him. It is another piece of him that helps me stay strong."

In the Buddhist tradition, giving away objects as opposed to words is characterized differently. When approaching death, one is advised to sever any attachments that can keep people alive because they cannot let go of something. That something may be a feeling, a person or an object. In the words of Buddhist master Sogyal Rinpoche:

> The ideal way for a person to die is having given away everything, internally and externally, so that there is as little as possible yearning, grasping, and attachment for the mind at that essential moment to latch on to. So before we die we should try to free ourselves of attachment to all our possessions, friends and loved ones. We cannot take anything with us, so we should make plans to give away all our belongings beforehand as gifts or offerings to charity.[10]

Let go of things and of people, thing by thing, person by person, so that you can leave the world free.

The Tibetan *lama* we met earlier, Gehlek Rimpoche, tells the story of the attachment of his master in *Good Life, Good Death*. Two of his master's students were old men in failing health who were eager to die and decided on a date for death with their master, a practice reserved for those with a highly developed capacity for meditation. The men began to sever their attachments, gave away their possessions and made arrangements. One man died "on schedule." The other did not. The master went to see his old student on the brink of death to find out what was getting in the way of letting go. The student said that he had all the signs of death, but then they suddenly reversed themselves. It was painful for him. Suddenly, the master noticed that his student was wearing a new shirt that had been given to him two days before.

He told his student that he liked the shirt and wanted it. The student protested. He too liked the shirt very much and was not anxious to give it away. His master insisted, threatening that the two would have nothing to do with each other if he did not get the shirt. The old man, not wanting to lose his master, took the shirt off. The master ripped it into pieces before his student's eyes, and his student died soon after. The attachment to a shirt was keeping him alive.[11]

For Buddhists, severing attachments is their way of taking care of unfinished business. Gehlek Rimpoche said that one of the last times he saw his father, his father said, "When I die, I will not come to you to seek help. I hope you can achieve the same thing."[12]


A few years after Alyssa died, my aunt Diane told me that she was mailing me a package, and I should be on the lookout for it. It was around the time of my birthday, but we don't usually exchange gifts. I couldn't imagine what it was. I opened a small curved navy silk box, and in it was a set of pearl and diamond earrings. I called my aunt to thank her for the thoughtful and unexpected present.

"They were Alyssa's. I bought them for her for her wedding. That was the last time she wore them."

Suddenly the gift took on another dimension. It felt odd to own something of beauty worn last on the day of a wedding that joined two people never fated for marital success, kind of like wearing the wedding ring of a woman who got divorced. And there was also the more pressing issue of Alyssa's death. I have an ivory pin of my paternal grandmother and a gold chain that once belonged to my husband's grandmother. I have a pearl bracelet from my husband's late aunt. I think of each of these women in a very personal way when I wear something that they wore. They are badges of honor and memory. But Alyssa died too young to be bequeathing jewelry. I hesitated to put the earrings on, knowing their history. But when I finally put them on and looked in the mirror and realized that I was carrying a piece of Alyssa with me, it felt good. It felt redemptive. The thought that they would have sat lonely in a drawer somehow made Alyssa seem farther away. She is closer now.

Inanimate objects are not the only items to be dispensed with at the death of a loved one. As I get older and think about what I want to leave behind, I've been thinking a lot more about my charitable giving. It's one of the few tangible ways to keep doing acts of goodness even when I'm no longer around, something that can have an impact now and beyond. And even if I might have been stingy in this life at times, I may be able to make up for it with some little last minute generosity. In Hebrew, the word for charity is *tzedaka*; *tzedaka* is not about goodness, it is about justice, which is what the word means. I might feel good about giving a few quarters to a homeless person who puts out a hand, but that is not creating a more just society. In the words of Percy Bysshe Shelley: "No man has a right to monopolize more than he can enjoy." Being a member of a universal family means equalizing the financial playing field between the haves and the have-nots. I heard this sentiment from a young successful businessman whose wife was pregnant with their first child: "I give 11 percent of what I make. I do it because I really believe that it doesn't belong to me. When you change the way that you think about money, it becomes a pleasure giving it all away. It's made my life a lot more whole."

I know that at times I've held on to money in this life, but I am not going to have any need for a wallet where I'm going. And the good news is that if I don't have a purse in the next life then I never have to clean it, and if I no longer have a wallet and keys then it's impossible to lose them in the next life. Now that's something to look forward to.

Endowing a charitable gift avoids a problem that the book of Ecclesiastes points to when discussing the difficulties of legacy giving. You work hard your whole life and leave money behind for the benefit of others, but you don't know what will happen to that nest egg when you hand it over:

> For a man may do his work with wisdom, knowledge and skill, and then he must leave all he owns to someone who has not worked for it. . . . What does a man get for all the toil and anxious striving with which he labors under the sun?[13]

You do not even get the assurance that what you worked for will be well spent if you don't use it all yourself. At least when you designate a charity of choice in your will, you do know where the money is going, and you do know that it will be a signature of what you cared about in this life.

Woody Allen once said, "It is impossible to experience one's own death objectively and still carry a tune." True, true. It is a challenge. It's hard to sing when you're dying. But it's not hard to think of ultimate words. They come naturally. Ordinary people who don't invent cures for diseases or write remarkable poetry can achieve immortality within their families with an ethical will. It is a document written by the dying containing life lessons, suggestions, recommendations and advice born of a lifetime of wisdom and experience. Ethical wills can take many forms, and they sure beat rehearsing your own funeral.

The ethical will is generally regarded as an ancient gift of the Hebrew Bible, and its significance transferred to the New Testament in the book of John.[14] It is traced back to Genesis 49, where Jacob gathered his many sons and gave them each a blessing. One medieval commentator believed that Jacob's blessings were a euphemism for "curses," such were Jacob's harsh recriminations. Jacob tried both to summarize the character of his sons and make predictions based upon this information that would challenge and grow their leadership. After all, these were not only his sons; they were future Israelite leaders whose progeny would become a nation. Jacob's last words were there to share a stunning truth from a man who had little to lose. Perhaps if he finally said what needed to be said to his family, Jacob's own vision for the future of his tribe would be realized.

We want last words to be words of peace and family unity. Such words help us remember the dead with kindness and compassion. People who leave this world with sharp words leave an indelible mark, an emotional scar that can never be removed. The words, repeated in our memories, bite again and again. But harmony can be a false god when there are life messages that are more messy and uncomfortable but that must, nonetheless, get expressed. In the words of a friend, "My father used to have a beard until his mother lay on her deathbed and told him to shave it off. He hasn't had one since."

Many regard the entire book of Deuteronomy as Moses' ethical will, his farewell address of advice and often acerbic words to a nation he had led for forty years as they transitioned from desert wanderers to stable homesteaders in the Promised Land. Their holy shepherd was not permitted to cross the Jordan River and accompany them. All he had to offer was a review of their time together, some recommendations for the next stop and some last words of preparation to mentor them for the difficulties ahead that he would not share. In Hebrew, the Latin word "Deuteronomy" is rendered as "*devarim,*" which means "words" or "things." The semantic connection is not incidental. Words are things; they have weight and heft and impact. Words have consequences. Moses' ethical will was loaded with the weight of accountability, accusation and criticism.

A medieval French biblical commentator believed that Moses' farewell speech was actually given as a rebuke. Ancient rabbis, commenting on Moses' decision to part this way, said that there are four reasons why people censure and chastise people on their deathbeds. I paraphrase and contemporize:

First: When people criticize us during their lifetimes, they often repeat their points again and again. As a result, we stop paying attention. When the dying offer difficult advice with their last breath to those they leave behind, the message can be heard because of its finality. "I'm saying it once, and I'm not saying it again."

Second: The person being criticized usually experiences shame, but in a deathbed scene, the listener is able to get beyond the shame simply so that he can grasp the message and hold it tightly.

Third: The person facing criticism will not hold a grudge because these are the very last words of the dying and, therefore, will become part of the totality of the person's imprint.

Finally: The recipient will listen in order for the parting to happen in peace.[15] Words left unsaid, the difficult unfinished emotional business of relationships, can get in the way of ever healing properly. "She said what she meant. We had it all out. We know where we stand."

I had a hard time believing that people would intentionally leave critical last words, and I regarded the biblical narrative as more of a literary device than anything else. That is, until I spoke with Jessie. Jessie underwent many surgeries for what she calls "weird problems."

She was undergoing a hysterectomy at age forty-nine and was nervous about being put to sleep after reading about people who never woke up or who woke up in a persistent vegetative state. It didn't help that she had lost her father at a similar age. Jessie's daughter was fourteen and her son was in college at the time, and she wanted to leave behind last words for them in case something went wrong. She also had some choice words for her husband. It wasn't that she did not love them or have kind words or gratitude to share. She did. But she was also worried. Her daughter was young, and the letter she left her had generic advice, but Jessie was more concerned about her son. She wanted to leave him some relationship advice; she felt that he was not giving or trusting enough and that this would affect him in the future. Jessie also wanted her husband to know how hard it was for her to be left alone so much in their marriage. Her husband is, in her words, a wonderful and giving physician, whose patients cannot stop talking about how remarkable he is. They joke that he must never be at home, and Jessie couldn't agree more. He isn't. She needed to let him know just how much this had impacted her life. She carried a lot of resentment for a long time, even though she was confident he truly loved her.

She wrote each of them a handwritten letter: "That's the only way I would do something like this, since handwriting is a part of you." Her letters were not long, maybe one page double-sided. She wasn't leaving behind a magnum opus, as she called it. She made them just long enough to say what she needed to say. Each started, "If you're reading this, it means I'm not around right now . . ." She told a close friend about the letters and tasked her with their delivery, should it be necessary. She left them in envelopes in her file cabinet.

Jessie's operation went smoothly, so smoothly, in fact, that she actually forgot all about the letters for years. One day, years later, as she was frantically looking through her files for something else, she came across them. Jessie reread them and agreed with everything she had written. By that time her son had gotten married, his trust issues resolved, and her daughter had grown up fine. "And with my husband, nothing had changed," she said. You could almost hear the shrug of resignation in her voice.

"Then I ripped them up. I don't know why I did. I got rid of the letters. Later on I had brain surgery, and I didn't write anything. We even bought cemetery plots right before the brain surgery, but I must have been in a different place if I didn't write to them. There are still things I want to say to them now. Of course there are. My husband and I should both write things, especially now that there are grandchildren. I probably should put it in writing. I will. Now there are new things to tell them."

She contemplated why she ripped up her last words: they weren't last words anymore. Times had changed. They were not relevant. Maybe she was less afraid to die, or maybe she was more afraid to die and now no longer wanted to face the reality of last words.

In their book *Ethical Wills*, Jack Riemer and Nathaniel Stampfer describe this unusual genre:

> Parents would write a letter to their children in which they would try to sum up all that they had learned in life, and in which they would try to express what they wanted most for and from their children. They would leave these letters behind because they believed that the wisdom they had acquired was just as much part of the legacy they wanted to leave their children as were all the material possessions.[16]

In some instances, parents left ethical wills because they had few material possessions to pass on. What they could give, all they could give, were the riches of advice and life experience.

The authors make us aware both of how difficult it is to write an ethical will and how emotionally challenging it is to read one. Parents writing such letters have to review their own lives carefully and confront their failures as well as their achievements in order to distill their last thoughts into bite-sized lessons. Reducing decades of life into essential truths and zeroing in on what matters most is never easy. The process of writing such a document is first and foremost an introduction to the self. It is a time of reading life backward and writing life forward for those who live after you.

Now imagine you're on the other side of this epistle. As Riemer and Stampfer observe:

> There is a sense of being a voyeur, of eavesdropping on an intimate conversation, of reading a love letter from beyond. . . . There is a temptation, an almost irresistible one, for parents to try to persuade after death what they were unable to persuade during life. There is the temptation to repeat once more, to plead once more, and to impose a burden of guilt from the grave.[17]

We can hear the future bleating of a mother: "I am asking you for the very last time, please eat your green vegetables and wear a sweater when you go outside. Now that I'm dead, will you *finally* listen to me?" Or a father: "Remember to keep your home insurance up to date and to balance your checkbook. Oh, also, don't forget to make sure there is enough air pressure in your tires."

I spoke with Elliott, whose paternal grandfather's ethical will actually makes an appearance in Riemer and Stampfer's book. It's a simple will, Elliott said, but it is clear that the will is far-reaching and informs his life and the lives of his family members. "My parents had a handwritten copy of it hanging on the wall in the family room, and now a copy of it hangs in my family room." He has passed on copies of it to his married children. "Five years ago a cousin organized a get-together of cousins and kids, about seventy of us, for the seventy-fifth anniversary of the writing of the will." Wow. They had a party for the anniversary of a will. They've had several get-togethers over the years. The will brought the family together and keeps bringing them together.

On the bottom of the will, beneath his signature, Elliott's grandfather specified his wish that the will would be read regularly, and at least annually on the anniversary of his death. It was written in March of 1932 before William was about to undergo major surgery. At the time it was a hazardous operation, and he prepared the document in anticipation that he would not make it. The surgery was successful, and William actually lived for another seventeen years, dying in 1949. Elliott believes that his grandfather's wish was observed: his desires informed the way the family lived. "I see it in the house. I show it to people who come over to the house. There's no flowery language. The point is to instruct his children how to conduct themselves in their lives with regard to family and with regard to other people at work and in society." William may have understood a secret that some people miss: keep it short, and they will read it. "Everyone knows it backward and forward. People in my generation have really tried to internalize it." Having it hanging in his home means that it is part of Elliott's everyday landscape. "To me, the fact that it is handwritten makes me feel like I have a real connection to him. You can see the personality of the author, not only by the substance but also by the handwriting."

The will is written in the format of a letter to his "dear children." He begins by invoking how hard he worked to give his family food, shelter and an education and raise them "to lead an honest, clean and respectable life." There is a certain reciprocity of decency he was trying to communicate. By living a certain life and giving his children certain tools and models, William was showing them through his own life what he expected in exchange. He wanted them to be strict Sabbath observers, eat only kosher food and uphold Jewish tradition. "Take care of your mother because she's your best friend in the world." Elliott agrees. "My grandmother was a wonderful, warm person, and she was well loved. That was easy."

It was important for William to tell his children to be honest in their commercial and social undertakings. "Never consider yourself better than the next man." This value was reinforced by his insistence that no one insult anyone else and that his children "talk and treat people kindly." In particular, William wanted his children to love one another: "Keep together; be friendly with one another. The will implied that the family was close and that good behavior was expected." William had six children, and, in Elliott's description, "The siblings really did love each other."

William closed his will by asking that his children pass along what he called his fatherly advice to the next generation, believing that if his children followed his advice, God would help them. I asked Elliott how everyone was doing in this large family in light of William's wishes. "The family always supported one another. There really was no conflict. No negative stuff." William gave this family the glue to avoid dramas and upsets that tear some families asunder. With a will this influential, I wondered if anyone else in Elliott's family had written an ethical will. Did Elliott have one? No. There were no other wills. "Why tinker with something that works? I interact with my kids, showing them by example how to live one's life. One of the things I do tell them is to be honest with yourself and with others. Tell the truth and communicate. I haven't really thought about doing something like this." It seems that William's will is *the* family will. Its advice is good and sensible, and Elliott feels, at heart, that he has nothing to add. His grandfather's ethical will produced decent human beings.

In the sixteenth century, Rabbi Abraham Horowitz, living in Poland, wrote an ethical will for his son, who wrote a commentary with emendations and his own thoughts on his father's will: on raising children, maintaining one's integrity, and the role of money, study and community in one's life. It became, in effect, his own ethical will, which he passed down to yet another generation. His son then wrote a commentary on *his* father's will. All three wills were published together. All gave the writer a chance to share the cumulative wisdom of three generations of one family who interpreted and internalized what the generation before wanted from their lives. Even so, an ethical will can only suggest. It cannot demand. It certainly cannot enforce.

I was learning how recipients of an ethical will used them and also wanted to see if the process of writing one would have an emotional impact. As an observer, I joined a workshop that was part of a five-day leadership development program in Colorado. The participants were uniformly successful and had been carefully selected from a pool of willing candidates who wanted to improve their leadership skills and deepen their values and commitments. This was their first encounter with one another across a two-year commitment, and the ethical will seminar was the last group exercise after a week of study and shared experiences. There was a freshness and an openness in the room. They were ready.

Before participants came to the retreat they were sent a document with questions to structure their ethical wills. They were asked in advance to think about the questions and, if they wanted to, to formulate answers. The desired format was a letter to someone they care about and to whom they want to leave their legacy. Usually it is designated for children, but not everyone in the group was married or had children. According to the directions, facilitators were to ask the participants "to write a letter to their children (or future children), or to those whom they will leave material possessions, or to those they hope they have influenced in some fashion, explaining to them what they hold important in life, and what they would like them to learn and to remember." The facilitator's role was "to create space and conditions for thoughtful writing time." Participants were given about an hour to write, with the understanding that they would most likely not finish the exercise in that amount of time but would have made a solid start.

Those in the group were told before the retreat that the purpose of the exercise was to provide closure to their learning and "translate the learning into concrete and relevant terms" by thinking about their own identity and values, how they planned to strengthen and transmit those values and the legacy they wished to leave. The workshop was divided into three parts: preparation, writing and discussion.

We got to the writing stage, and I expected people to walk out of the conference-room setting to soak up the inspiration of a magnificent Colorado afternoon. It had been raining intermittently, and drops of water dripped from the rounded leaves of Aspen birches. Wildflowers carpeted the hills, and it seemed altogether the perfect place to contemplate life's heavier questions. But instead, every participant sat in the large windowless basement hotel room, scribbling furiously, like the overachieving test-takers they were. Still, near the end of the hour there was some restlessness and whispering. It seemed hard to sustain the degree of intensity required for the exercise for long stretches of time. The group needed a psychic break. That break came in the form of Casey, the petite facilitator and one of the retreat's organizers, who was ready to have a meta-conversation on the process of writing the will and give people the opportunity to reflect on what they were doing and all of its emotional resonances. The facilitators were given a "script" of possible questions in advance to structure the exercise's debriefing:

- What was the experience of writing like for you? How did it feel?
- What was most challenging about this exercise? Why?
- How did you decide what you wanted to include in your ethical will?

- How do you translate these principles into your own life? How do you make these commitments visible to the outside world?
- Did anything you learned or experienced this week affect what you wrote?
- What additional things might you do to live out the values you have articulated for yourself?

Take a group of leaders, ask them a question and then sit back. Most leaders I know are talkers. They had a lot to say when Casey asked, "What did you feel doing this exercise?"

Holly sat at the front of the room and opened the conversation. She slid almost immediately into a puddle of feelings: "It's really hard. . . . It's sad. It's hard to contemplate a life where you're not here, especially if you have young children." She began to cry and then shrugged off the tears to continue. "Maybe this is just me speaking because I'm so self-centered." She laughed and brought a little relief to the room. Then she breathed in to control the emotional outpour about to come: "I lost my dad when I was so young. I think how precious it would have been if my father had left this for me. He died so young, and I don't know why, having gone through that experience myself, I didn't think about doing this before for my own kids." At this, she cried harder. Everyone sat in silence. Holly did not take herself seriously, but in thinking about what she wished she had from her own father, she realized that her words would be taken seriously one day. One day, her daughter may clench the piece of paper she was writing and read it in tears, holding on to her in some very visceral way.

Attention moved from one cluster of the room to another as people offered small pieces of what they wrote or the feelings behind the words. Some people in the seminar did not want to share, and many felt that this was too public a setting for this kind of exercise. One young social entrepreneur felt that he was not old enough to write an ethical will. His life was just starting out and he had, in his words, a lot more mistakes to go. He and his wife were just beginning a family. Instead, he wanted to go back home and do the exercise with his parents, and he even asked the group to submit questions to ask their parents or aging relatives.

The group had been dry-eyed for twenty minutes until Casey decided to move the conversation along with another leading question: "Why did you include what you did in your letter?"

Sylvie, a beautiful Latin American woman, brought the emotions back into the room and told the group that she wrote her letter to her three kids and wanted it to be read often, not just at the end. She was weeping heavily as she reflected on the pain of the exercise. She wanted her children to read the letter when they found themselves facing challenges they thought they could not handle. As she said this, she began to cry again, knowing that her three boys would have troubled times ahead when she would not be there to help them through the darkness. At the same time, she sounded insecure about her own choices, questioning if she had made the correct decisions. "I worry that we're surrounded by false mirrors, and we think we're better than we are. I want them, more than anything, to put themselves in another person's shoes without losing their own identities, through being strong. I want them to bring light to whoever is around them." And as she said these last words, her voice took on greater confidence.

Like a few others in the room, Sylvie revealed the personal insecurity of writing an ethical will. How do you know you've got it right? How do you know if you're living the lessons you want to pass on? Will those who come after you see through this letter and come to the conclusion to do as you say but not as you do? Are we surrounding ourselves with Sylvie's false mirrors? Are we authentic?

Casey took advantage of the silence to ask one quick question before time ran out. "Do you think you are any different than you were a week ago?" Tom implied that it was not so much the content but behaviors that show the differences from one week to the next: "I was thinking about writing this letter before I got here. Really. But then I thought it would be morbid to think about my demise and so I didn't write it. But this wasn't depressing. It actually felt like a normal activity, and it made this whole idea of death more real."

Sally had not really spoken up yet but now she added her two cents in support of Tom's idea. She is a trustee for someone else's estate and sees how kids really do wonder if they have done what their parents wanted with their money and their lives. "I think when you write a letter like this, it gives your kids absolution. It sets them free. They understand what you want. They don't spend their lives guessing." Sally's words struck a chord. Josh said, "I love the word 'absolution.' Until you just said that I didn't think about how an ethical will can liberate people of all the guesswork. That really means something to me."

The hour was getting late, and we had almost used up the time that we'd been allotted, when Stacy spoke up: "When I was young we lost a close friend of my father's very suddenly. We all knew that so much was left unsaid. I don't think we should hold things back. My kids always know what I think because I don't want to write down my thoughts and then tuck them away for a lifetime. This was a good exercise to think about how to live every day. I'm not saving it all up for one piece of paper."

Casey took the floor back and asked the group if they had any questions before they ended the session. Sylvie asked Casey if she had done this exercise herself.

"I've done it several times," Casey replied. "I've watched this process for twenty-two years of retreats, and my own thoughts have evolved over time."

Sylvie prodded her: "Do you save the old ones so that you and others can see how you've evolved?"

- 239 -

This introduced a new concept to the group. As we change and evolve, do our letters change and evolve? Should we be saving each copy of our ethical wills, so that those after us can see how we've changed? Sylvie added, "I think it would be interesting for those we leave behind to see how we've grown and changed. Maybe other people will really understand that life is a process from us."

Casey understood Sylvie's logic, but it did not reflect her own thinking. "No. That's not the kind of person I am. I want my last version to be *the* version because it reflects who I am now."

No one else had a question or a concluding thought. They had been sitting in the same room for what seemed like hours, and as Casey thanked the group for the session, people began to rise from their seats and stretch their legs the way that people do when they've just come off a long flight. Having been with the group all week, I sensed a change, a change in the physical closeness of the group as they spoke with one another, a change in the intensity of the conversation and the expectation of meaning. There was a density, an emotional humidity, that made everything feel slower and foggier. The group was quiet and pensive as they left the room. The banalities of break-time conversations were not appropriate to the thickness in the air. Hesitatingly, they left the conference room and went into the hall, another, different space. They had just begun the process of writing an ethical will. The first stab at it was sobering, but it had helped them understand that a happier ending is one where one's values are clearly articulated, even if the process is heart-wrenching and heavy.

Now they had to reenter the world and live their words before they became last words.

*Chapter Eight*

# The Last Apology

When I think back to the day my search for a better death began, I keep reliving the image of Diane and Roy saying their final "sorrys" as Alyssa's body was wheeled out of her apartment. All the grief resurfaced. I see in my mind's eye the friends and relatives standing at the edge of Alyssa's grave and depositing flowers and apologies on top of her casket as the dirt falls loosely from the walls. And I am standing there again, in the rain, silenced by the solemnity and finality of the moment.

We all know someone who went to the grave bitter about a "sorry" never given or received. After death, those open wounds have little chance of healing. For the living, they can fester for decades and become emotionally paralyzing. It takes courage to realize when to forgive and how before time runs out. But after it runs out, the well of sadness can be deep and vast. And I began to understand the confusion and despair when we can no longer be on the receiving end of forgiveness. One "sorry" does not repair every problem, but it may diminish distance in some relationships. Out of all the last words we consider saying, the most important two may be "I'm sorry." The three most important words may be "I forgive you." When we lose that opportunity, we might spend the rest of our lives in regret.

Esther says sorry to Joe all the time, but he is no longer alive to forgive her. Esther met her husband, Big Joe, in a local bar when she was nineteen. Too young to drink, she went there to dance and play the bowling games. A petite blond, short of five feet, Esther was on the rebound and attracted to Joe's kind, gentle manner, wrapped in his hulking six-foot size. Like Esther, Joe loved to play the bowling machines. They dated for about five years because Esther was busy working, and her parents were unhappy that she was in an interfaith relationship. So were his. While neither set were religiously observant, they were culturally affiliated and they let their feelings be known. Esther's family spoke to her about it. Her sister noodled her into rethinking the relationship, but it did not work. Esther and Joe were in love. They finally married without their parents' blessing in a civil ceremony in a courthouse. Esther's boss threw her a small wedding party. They launched their lives together and made their marriage work. When Big Joe died, the couple had been married for forty years.

Joe's death was a shock to Esther and her three sons. Joe's golfing buddies took him to the hospital on a Monday when he looked unwell. By Friday he was dead.

No one knew that Joe was sick. He enjoyed life. He was an athlete and was generally in good health, despite the onset of diabetes. Joe traveled globally on business and was a work-hard, play-hard type of guy. He used his downtime to play golf and cards. He was a big guy, and when he got bigger, Esther had tried unsuccessfully to get him to diet. He never told anyone when he was unwell. Esther finally started accompanying him to his physicals because he would never tell her what the doctors said. Most likely he developed sepsis after suffering with gallstones, not something he had to die for. No autopsy was performed, so the family will never really know what happened. What Esther does know is that on Monday Big Joe was in her life and by Friday he wasn't.

On Wednesday of the week Joe died, the local hospital that admitted him transferred him to a larger teaching hospital. He was in excruciating pain, and they wanted to get to the bottom of it. By Friday, all of his organs were shutting down. Close to forty people came to see him off. Esther reminisces: "The last day there were so many people with me that they had to give us a private room. They emptied the physicians' lounge. I think we were all in shock." A pompous surgeon came in who claimed to have seen a woman in her thirties in similar condition who, in his words, had a whole life ahead of her. Joe was not in that position. "The surgeon made it sound as if Joe's life just wasn't worth fighting for," Esther says with bitterness. Esther's daughter-in-law was so outraged by the doctor's arrogance she said she would never be in the room with the man again.

Later that day, a more compassionate physician spoke to Esther. Esther did not shoo everyone out for the conversation. "I'm a very open person. I'm mouthy, and I have a lot of opinions. Whatever the doctor was going to say, he could say it in front of everyone."

The doctor's words were direct: "Joe is failing. He is starting to shut down, and you're going to have to make a decision."

Esther was nervous because she did not have the power of attorney and believed that she needed it to make the decision. Joe and she had never discussed the end. "We had no discussion of end of life anything." There was no medical directive. Joe was like 71 percent of Americans, according to a study done by the Pew Research Center. He did not have a living will.[1] Even when he was rushed to the hospital on

Monday, his family never believed he was going to die. He never said any last words on Tuesday or Wednesday. There were no teary "sorrys" or "goodbyes." Esther scrambled to get a lawyer friend involved for the necessary documentation. In the end she did not need it. She needed only to give the doctors permission to pull the plug. Joe was already brain dead. This was not a persistent vegetative state where the body could breathe on its own, waiting until the heart shut down. Joe was being kept alive but would never return to any real functioning.

"I was afraid that they would not honor our wishes since we were in a Catholic hospital. If we didn't do anything, he would linger. He would just linger. All I could think of was that if he didn't have the quality of life to do what he always loved, he would be miserable, and I wouldn't wish that on my worst enemy."

The head doctor said, "It's your decision."

"He looked at all of us—about two dozen," Esther continued, "and said that it didn't matter what religion we were; we all came from Abraham, Isaac and Jacob. We're all the same under the skin, so no matter what religious path we choose to take, he said, 'I will do whatever you want me to do.'"

She made the decision to terminate Joe's life. "A member of the clergy was there and my sons, my daughter-in-law, my grandchildren, some of our closest friends. We kept talking to him even after they pulled the plug. We started singing 'Hail to the Redskins,' and the next thing I knew, he was gone."

Big Joe was buried on a crisp, sunny day in October, weather that seemed too beautiful for an unexpected graveside burial. Esther read a poem she composed; she often wrote poems for family occasions. This would be her last to Joe. Friends were amazed that she had the composure, especially given the suddenness of it all. But Esther came from a Navy family. She said that she had never seen either of her parents cry. She was able to hold it together.

•   •   •

A few months later, Esther joined a bereavement group for women given through a local hospice. "We went through the guilt and the anger. We talked about not being touched, about being alone. We had a facilitator. All the widows kept talking about how much they loved their husbands, and the whole time I'm thinking, *What if I hadn't given the order to turn it off?* How could I play God and say, 'Well, he won't have his regular full life of what he enjoys'?" Esther worried that maybe she didn't love her husband as much as these other women loved theirs if it was so easy for her to pull the plug on Joe's life.

For the many years following Joe's death, Esther has apologized to Joe again and again. "I am the one who put an end to it all." She reviews that decision in her mind constantly; it has a stranglehold over her. "For that brief moment and since then, I have thought and thought and said and said and said to Joe in my mind and my heart, out loud, 'I am sorry.'"

I asked Esther if she would have made a different decision now that she lives with so much guilt. "I hope I didn't make the wrong decision. I think I made the right decision. I think Joe would say I made the right decision, I don't know. No one in the room said not to. Not even my sons. Not even the son who was closest to Big Joe."

I was stymied. If she believed she made the right decision, a decision that Joe would have made himself had he been able to, then why was she so tortured? Why did she constantly seek Joe's forgiveness? Esther answered my question haltingly. "I have never told anyone this before, but when I was making that decision, I was not only thinking about Joe. I was also thinking about myself. Keeping him alive would have changed my whole life, and I didn't want that life." She sought Joe's forgiveness for not being willing to sacrifice more of herself as a caregiver. She did not kill Joe, but she wanted a clearer conscience about her decision to end his life. Did she do this for him, or did she also pull the plug for herself?

> When I made that decision, I had to decide what my life would be. Don't think that thought didn't cross my mind—the idea of being a caregiver for someone forevermore was part of my decision. I'm not stupid. I know what was going in my head. . . . I can't get rid of this guilt so I will have to live with this for the rest of my life. I wonder. I wonder, *Could they have done something more?*

Esther believes that unresolved guilt comes with a forever price tag. Because we've known each other for years, I spoke to Esther about pursuing therapy to relieve some of the sting. Esther was uninterested. It almost felt as if she wanted to punish herself. Fiercely independent, she was not looking for pity or an easy way out. We talked about her saying "sorry" at the grave. She kept a journal for a while after Joe's death. He keeps coming back to her not only out of love but out of guilt, a guilt that cannot, in her mind, be removed without a proper apology to him. She whispers it or says it in her mind. I asked her if she thought writing a letter to him would take the guilt, resentment and "what-if-ness" of these shadows and externalize them, taking them outside herself and letting them go, creating a big helium balloon of sadness and letting it float far away. She told me she would think about it.

I was shocked by how few books and comprehensive guides for hospice patients and the dying include chapters or even a paltry sentence on the importance of forgiveness before death, let alone what to do with a "sorry" that would never be heard. There are few acts more rich with meaning than forgiveness at the end. Did no one outside of religion think of that?

Jewish tradition remedies Esther's tortured guilt impulse with ritual. If you need to apologize to someone who has already died, in Jewish law you can bring a quorum of people to the gravesite and apologize publicly. On the one hand, the person six feet under is not going to respond (and if he or she does, watch out). But on the other hand, the idea of verbalizing that which was previously unsaid in front of a makeshift community is one way of turning oneself inside out. The apology responds to an internal, unmet need for forgiveness by pulling it out of the self and making it public.

Death without forgiveness is regarded in most faiths as a spiritual omission of a high order. People should apologize to the dying in this lifetime for intentional hurt, *and* the dying must also confess their wrongdoing to leave the world with a clean slate. We might think of this as just words, and empty words for many, a pro forma kind of admission. Yet the need is there even when it goes unrecognized; maybe we only realize it when the chance goes away, the way that it did for Esther.

Christians and Muslims ritualize the act of forgiveness before one dies through prayer; saying "sorry" before death is the last act of Jews, who are supposed to follow a formula in the prayerbook but can say whatever they want if words escape them in the moment. One code of Jewish law from the sixteenth century discusses this with an almost humorous concern: namely, what if a person fails to confess because he is worried that once he confesses he will die? The confession, in his mind, will effectuate his death:

When death draws near, one is advised to confess. And we reassure him: "Many have confessed and then not died just as many have confessed and died." If he is unable to confess aloud, let him confess in his heart. If he does not know what to do we instruct him to say: "May my death be an expiation for all my sins." This is not done in the presence of women and children lest they cry and break his heart.[2]

Words won't kill you, but the tears of a weepy wife and kids just might.

Even if Esther were to bring her whole family to the cemetery where Joe is buried, he would still not respond, but the ritual might take the sting that haunts people like Esther and render it less powerful. She learned a lot about how to have a better death from Joe's death. As a result of Joe's experience, Esther made a living will and designated one of her sons to make the decision to end her life if she were unable make the decision herself. She wants to make sure that her children will really try to embody her wishes, in the way that she tried to embody Joe's, despite her own concerns. She understands too well the dangers of second-guessing. She knows that the decision haunts her and revisits her because *she* made it for Joe. She did not know exactly what he wanted. She could only approximate what she thought he would have wanted. And she knows now that part of a happy ending is not leaving others guessing because a decision that should have been theirs lodges in you and does not let you go.

"I really do believe that people who have died come back to you in your dreams," Esther told me. "When you are feeling really, really low they come to you. My parents come to me in my dreams. Joe comes to me in my dreams sometimes. I want to hold on to him in my dream. And then he goes."

Esther made the need for one last "sorry" very clear. She helped me contemplate the nature of forgiveness and what we are doing when we say sorry or when we forgive, especially at the end of life. I'll never forget a sermon I heard more than twenty years ago that began with one question: is it harder to say sorry or harder to forgive? I think the latter wins hands down in any emotional competition. Mastering the art of forgiveness feels at times like scaling a mountain.

I've always been awed and surprised by people who forgive those who murdered their children when they try to stay an execution. They somehow have a compassion gene that outweighs a justice gene. It seems a spiritual stretch I'm incapable of making, but then again, I have not been tested the way others have. I'm awed by the Christian embrace of forgiveness and that the central figure of Christianity is a person who died in heroic, tragic circumstances to seek forgiveness for the living. Jesus created a remarkably high bar in modeling forgiveness, and he helped the rest of the world understand what we give others when we forgive them: we give them life.

Research demonstrates that people who forgive based on moral principle are found to be both healthier than those who forgive for the sake of obligation alone and better able to manage the emotional price of insult or hurt.[3] When forgiving easily is part of your spiritual makeup, you wake up more healthy each day. You probably sleep a whole lot better, especially if we're talking about eternal sleep.

The Reverend Martin Luther King Jr. believed that forgiveness is the one true watershed that allows ultimate peace, and he said as much when he wrote "Loving Your Enemies" while in jail for committing nonviolent acts of civil disobedience during the Montgomery bus boycott. In a church in Alabama on Christmas of 1957, King said, "We must develop and maintain the capacity to forgive. Whoever is devoid of the power to forgive is devoid of the power to love." This forgiveness begins not with the one who offends but with the one who is offended. Only the victim can initiate lasting forgiveness:

> The forgiving act must always be initiated by the person who has been wronged, the victim of some great hurt, the recipient of some tortuous injustice, the absorber of some terrible act of oppression. The wrongdoer may request forgiveness. . . . But only the injured

neighbor, the loving father back home, can really pour out the warm waters of forgiveness.[4]

The implications of this for deathbed forgiveness are astounding. If we have been offended by a dying person, it is up to *us* to provide the opportunity to forgive by granting our forgiveness, even when it is not requested.

Yet if people are not ready to grant forgiveness, forcing or expecting it may only disappoint and deepen the rift. Harriet Lerner in *The Dance of Connection* understands that a relationship can hit a crisis point, where we need an apology or need to say what we feel, but the relationship has never benefited from that kind of openness or safety. A deathbed is usually no place to start. She reminds us that we have to be cautious when expecting a dramatic apology or even offering one that the recipient may not be ready to hear:

> Sometimes voicing our thoughts and feelings shuts down the lines of communication, diminishes or shames another person or makes it less likely that two people can hear each other or stay in the same room. Nor is talking always a solution. We know from personal experience that our best intentions to process a difficult issue can move a situation from bad to worse.[5]

In certain ways, the death of others with unresolved forgiveness issues should prompt us to take the daily attempt at forgiveness more seriously. We can only control ourselves. We can offer forgiveness but not force someone else to accept it. We can accept that others make mistakes, even costly mistakes, and learn to live with them. Forgiveness is not only an act; it is an attitude that we carry with us about relationships.

In Jewish tradition, there is a prayer that many read before going to sleep that grants forgiveness randomly and comprehensively:

Master of the Universe, I forgive anyone who angered or troubled me or wronged me, whether to my person, my finances, my dignity or any other offense, whether it was done under coercion or done as an act of will, accidentally or intentionally, with words or with actions, in this life or another. . . . May the words of my heart find favor before You, God, My Rock and Redeemer.

A twentieth-century scholar commended anyone who said this prayer, believing it would extend one's life. It might not guarantee a longer life, but it might help with the quality of your life. Imagine all those nights spent in bed, ulcers growing bigger as you stew over an insult. The forgiveness habit is both lifelong and has long-life dividends.

I wondered how Reverend King would have managed had he been in Simon Wiesenthal's place. In his book *The Sunflower*, which is part autobiography, part fiction, Wiesenthal writes of his experience as a concentration camp victim who was called away from his work detail to visit an SS man dying in a hospital bed. The Nazi called Wiesenthal over to confess his sins and ask for absolution from the Jews. He longed to share his experiences and beg for atonement, but he did not know that there were any Jews left. When Wiesenthal appeared, the murderer was contrite: "I know that what I am asking is almost too much for you, but without your answer I cannot die in peace."[6] Wiesenthal struggled with his conscience. On the one hand, here was a dying man, and Wiesenthal's acquittal could help him ease the intensity of his pain without anyone else knowing. On the other hand, the SS man "was confessing his crime to a man who perhaps tomorrow must die at the hands of these murderers." Wiesenthal looked out the window, where his eye caught sight of German graves marked with sunflowers. One apology was not going to stop the heinous behavior of thousands of other unrepentant German soldiers. Wiesenthal looked at the man and, without a word, left the room. Maybe Reverend King would have forgiven the Nazi. Maybe not.

Reflecting on the incident decades later, Wiesenthal wondered if he should have stayed in the room and forgiven the Nazi. He put this question to human rights activists, members of the clergy, philosophers, writers and psychiatrists, who all had something to say about his action and his judgment. Some believed that forgiveness, if sincere, must always be granted, especially because in this case it would harm no one and help the dying man leave this world with solace. The majority believed that Wiesenthal had no right to grant forgiveness on behalf of others, of an entire people, as a singular voice. This reasoning drove Wiesenthal's own strongest instinct. Had the dying man recovered, it is not clear that he would have condemned or stopped any future atrocities. His contrition was likely the result of his situation. Wiesenthal's deathbed forgiveness scene prompts a difficult and niggling question: what does forgiveness fix?

Essayist and novelist Cynthia Ozick responded to Wiesenthal's conundrum with a firm sense of limitation. She believes that blanket forgiveness invalidates a victim's experiences, "blurring over suffering and death," obscuring the past. "It cultivates sensitiveness towards the murderer at the price of insensitiveness toward the victim."[7] The very last of Wiesenthal's respondents believes the fact that Wiesenthal was still reviewing this incident in his mind with such intensity means that his morality was still intact.

Even if we cannot forgive Wiesenthal's dying man, we can appreciate the fact that he asked for forgiveness. Often a "sorry" is a pass, a card we collect in the board game of life that sets us free. Yet we can acknowledge the chutzpah of the SS man's request while still expecting no less of him. A Nazi who could not apologize with his last breath would have learned nothing. The apology was a shadowy grasp

in darkness for a glimmer of redemption, a redemption largely unde-
served. It was met with the ambiguity of silence.

In these seeds of grace or rejection, we begin to understand the power
and limitation of the deathbed forgiveness. Wiesenthal could not
forgive a man for the sin committed against others, but nor could he
deny forgiveness either. He walked away. But in a relationship where
the dying focus their forgiveness on the individual who alone was offended, it becomes harder to walk away. No one is pretending that the
acts of hurt we inflict on one another will cease to exist, but instead
these insults are somehow pushed aside to a spot where they are no
longer a constant obstacle to love. "When there has been emotional
conflict or turmoil within families, the impending death of a family
member can be an opportunity for healing," writes Ira Byock. "What
would your mother most have wanted to see happen before she died?
If the answer is that she would have liked to see you or your father or
sister forgive each other for past hurts, consider what a gift doing so
would be to her."[8] In this instance, the apology is not directly offered
either by the person dying or to that person but between otherwise estranged family members or friends. Byock contends that this can help
the person who is dying leave this world with greater equanimity and
actually be a form of permission to leave, since the anguish of an unresolved or openly hostile relationship can be an ever-present obstacle
to dying in peace. It is a different type of exit strategy, one with many
spiritual ramifications. One small "sorry" can make a world of difference to the living and the dying.

Jackie will tell you that it's true: one small "sorry" *can* make a universe of difference to the living and the dying. Jackie grew up close to

her maternal grandparents, particularly her grandmother. Her grandfather was a lawyer and a judge, a stern man by her account: "My grandfather was more strong-willed than anyone you've ever met." She says this as fact, not as speculation.

Jackie's mother had an older brother who died at age two of pneumonia. When her mother's younger brother, Austin, was born there seemed to be instant pressure on him to be the older son his father lost, someone to carry on the name. Jackie's theory is that her grandfather wanted to make Austin into someone he never wanted to be. "My grandfather and my uncle did not see eye-to-eye. He pressured him to be everything: devoted, religious, professional, successful. He grew up in a household where he felt constricted and fought it his whole life." As soon as he was able, at the age of eighteen, Austin ran away to Canada to escape both the draft and his father. From that point on, Jackie's grandfather did not speak to his son . . . for twenty years.

I asked Jackie to describe her uncle: does she know him and have a relationship with him? "Oh God, yes. Austin is a character. He has always been rebellious. He's an artist who had no interest whatsoever in the professional world or in religion. He's always been anti-establishment, maybe just anti-anything and certainly against everything that my grandfather wanted him to be." We talk more about how Austin might have become rebellious, when Jackie asks out loud, "Did my grandfather make him like that? I don't know. Austin always thought my grandfather was very hard on him and had unrealistic expectations of what he could become."

After spending time in Canada, Austin moved to London, where he has lived ever since, an inconvenient ocean away. He moved to the other side of the world, more and more steps away from his childhood home. He married a woman from yet another country and another faith, taking a few more steps away, and had a daughter with her. He then divorced. In all the years, his father made no contact with him. He had no interest in Austin or his granddaughter. Austin became a photographer of the downtrodden of the world and now lives on a council estate, the English euphemism for "government housing." Jackie visited him there and was surprised to find brightly colored walls and plants all over his flat, just like his mother's home. "That's my grandmother in him. I saw pieces of her all over his apartment. She was the moon and the stars to everyone. She actually loved Austin for who he was and accepted him." Jackie's grandmother would visit Austin alone in London without telling her husband. Jackie knew that her grandmother kept the relationship hidden. "Maybe it was a don't-ask-don't-tell policy because my grandfather knew she was going away. He never forbade her. He didn't tell anyone else not to have ties with Austin. He just never spoke about him. Nothing."

How do you heal a scar that is decades old? First you have to name it. In *The Process of Forgiveness*, William Meninger acknowledges that it is important to think not only about who needs to be forgiven but also what we are asking forgiveness for: the very specific hurts and wounds that have not healed over time. We must acknowledge the extent of the injuries: "We have to see what they have done to our trust, our sense of justice, our self-esteem, and our ability to relate freely to our world." An act that hurt others years or decades ago has repercussions that we may never know or fully come to terms with because we are afraid to confront the pain that we caused. But once we face death closely, there is little to be afraid of anymore.

We can stop denying the hurt that we created with all the tentacles of that hurt that spread and poisoned the very lifeblood of another person, a friend or family member. We can take responsibility for the pain. To end this life better, we must. Meninger asks us to apologize, however, only when it is sincere and when the apology is able to capture in the very real and particular way what the dying have done wrong. "It means we can no longer deny what happened. We no longer attempt to explain it away or try to understand the other person and why the 'hurt' might have occurred. We no longer pretend it didn't happen, trivialize its effect on us, or try to forget it. It means we look at the hurt and its effect on us; we look at what our lives would have been without the hurt."[9] Contemplating what life would have been like without that hurt in some ways intensifies the anguish, but it also helps us get to the other side of the relationship.

Somewhere along the line, the tension thawed for Jackie's grandfather. He developed Parkinson's at a relatively young age and lived with it for decades. There was a slow progression to his illness, but when it got particularly bad, he moved to be nearer his daughter and her family. As Jackie described it, life suddenly took an odd turn:

> One day Grandpa decided he was not going to live forever so he said to my grandmother, "I think I have to see Austin." He had not talked to him for probably twenty years. It was really Austin's whole adult life. My grandmother contacted him and said, "I need you to do this for me." Austin had no money so they had to pay for his ticket, but he came. He did not say no.

The change in Jackie's otherwise stubborn grandfather took the whole family by surprise. But nationwide studies of older adults do show a change in attitude as we age when it comes to forgiveness. Forgiving others helps psychological well-being as people approach death and try to come to terms with the past and their own mistakes. Seniors who expect others to ask for forgiveness are more likely to experience psychological distress than those who can forgive unconditionally. And if people believe that God forgives them, they are less likely as they age to need the forgiveness of other people.[10] Jackie's grandfather was an old religious man in poor health. Could he have finally realized that he needed to make peace for himself, if not for his son? In Jackie's words, "I'm not sure if they felt death was imminent, even though my grandfather was already sick. There was happiness in finding each other and a relationship with some life left still to live."

Jackie found the reconciliation astounding. "My grandfather was a shrivel of a man by then. He was in a wheelchair. From that point onward, he and Austin made peace. They fell back together again. Grandpa died not long after. Austin told me he had already said goodbye in his own way. Sadly, they were in each other's lives for a very short time." Father and son could not make up for lost time. Austin's life was shaped by his father's rejection; last-minute attempts to jump-start a failing relationship could not sweeten the bitter water under the bridge. But such attempts are better than taking every last bit of resentment to the grave.

There was one other person profoundly affected by the break: Jackie's grandmother. She did not share her husband's harsh feelings and found the situation utterly heartbreaking. She had lost one son, and for most of Austin's life, she lost another. Although she made genuine attempts to keep the family together, Austin was still an ocean away. "They hurt each other so much, and they wouldn't fix it," Jackie says, still with disbelief. "Given all of the wounds they created in each other's lives, it is amazing that they found it within themselves to speak before he died."

•　　•　　•

$B$ut they did speak. Maybe the door to repentance does stay open, even a crack. In *Why Forgive?* the pastor and social critic Johann Christoph Arnold writes that no act closes that door, however cruel or despairing. A "sorry" does not minimize the act, for Arnold, but it is there to rehabilitate the relationship. "Forgiveness does not mean ignoring what has been done or putting a false label on an evil act. It means, rather, that the evil act no longer remains as a barrier to the relationship."[11]

Not everyone sees the open door of forgiveness. If you close that door too tightly, sorrow follows. The Todd family door appeared locked. Michael Todd, the chief constable of the Greater Manchester (UK) Police, scanned numerous websites to learn how to take his life.[12] A few days later, he texted his wife, Carolyn, that he was in a dark place and had destroyed himself. He wanted to end it all. Only days before, Carolyn had confronted him about an affair, and he confessed. He told Carolyn that he had been ill for a long time and had enough of life. At age fifty he was found dead on Mount Snowdon next to an empty gin bottle. He wrote one last text to his family: "I'm sorry for what I have done, forgive me in another life."

$W$hy wait for another life? Asking for forgiveness right before dying in this case seems odd, almost inappropriate. The one begging for forgiveness will not be around to receive it. And with forgiveness, this family may have been able to overcome the momentary darkness. The transactional aspect of forgiveness is sacrificed, perhaps because, in the mind of the penitent, the severity of the crime vitiates any chance he has for a pardon. In these small acts, a few words of contrition are the last offering of communication between the one who asks and the one who receives forgiveness. Only with his life did Michael Todd expect to pay the price for his wrongdoing. Nothing less would suffice. The "text" of forgiveness here was a last-ditch effort to reach beyond the chasm of death and plead for some degree of closeness or grace or understanding. But in Todd's mind the betrayal was actually unforgivable. He did not believe, in Arnold's words, that the door to forgiveness stays open even a crack. While it is true that he had to say he was sorry, *he* could not forgive himself and he imagined that others had closed that door too.

In this instance, Todd believed that only with his life could he replace that which he took from the world: trust. The depressed constable who ended it all did not understand that his death would not be a consolation for the damage and emotional havoc he created. It simply created more trauma, more ugliness for his wife, his friends and his children. Offering himself as a blemished sacrifice, Michael Todd preferred to die saying "sorry" than muster the bravery to live as a flawed person.

Austin's father, on the other hand, was prepared to face and confess a terrible mistake, allowing Austin a remaining sliver of peace once his father was gone. Austin could have said no, but in granting forgiveness he was giving up the right to hurt his father for hurting him. Carolyn's husband, however, left the hurt wide open. Carolyn may have forgiven him, but he will never know.

When it comes to saying "sorry" or hearing it, there is a significant lag time between the act and the acceptance. This distance often boils down to the difference between the cognitive or intellectual act of apologizing, which may take an instant, and the emotional readiness to integrate that apology into a relationship, which may take years. People often ask for forgiveness right after they've hurt someone or the offense becomes known. But the punch of this knowledge has to be digested and processed before the receiving party can ever really forgive. And that takes time. The problem with deathbed forgiveness is that we don't always have the time, or the one who needs to grant the forgiveness is not there to offer it. The suddenness of it all dazzles and confuses.

When the end is near for us or someone we love, and the bloated carcass of our egos has collapsed, it is time to put the hurt aside and to love. Saying "sorry" is an act of love. Forgiveness without a living path to redemption is hard to achieve, but sometimes it's all we have to offer. With our strength diminished at the end of life, love may be the only gift we have left to give. And "sorry" may be the only word we can say. And it may be enough.

*Chapter Nine*

# Learning from Grief

Happier endings are not just for those who leave us but for those who remain. Grieving well is highly cathartic. You weep for what you love, and it feels good to love that much. Winston Churchill once said, "If you go through hell, keep going." When you can grieve with the totality of yourself, then gratitude eventually conquers loss. You can look back on the life of a loved one and realize that the person, in some remarkable way, is still with you, an essence that remains with you in the emotional and spiritual residue left behind. The poet Philip Larkin captures the smoldering impact of grief in "If grief could burn out":

> *If grief could burn out*
> *Like a sunken coal,*
> *The heart would rest quiet,*

*The unrent soul*
*Be still as a veil;*
*But I have watched all night*
*The fire grow silent,*
*The grey ash soft:*
*And I stir the stubborn flint*
*The flames have left,*
*And grief stirs, and the deft*
*Heart lies impotent.*[1]

And for the moment, we are with Larkin in the middle of the night, stirring his pain, watching the ashes gather. Watching grief, almost as if it lies outside the self, does not make it go away. Grief lingers. When we grieve we mourn the loss of another and the piece of that other person who became part of us. We grieve a loss of ourselves. And when we are able to grieve fully, we can sometimes translate that grief later on into loving more fully, because death's intimacy was so close and painful.

In contrast, holding grief in can lead to emotional detachment from our warmest memories and reside within us as a very unhappy, unresolved ending. Ironically, people who grieve the loudest and cry the most at a funeral are often crying over a relationship that needed repair and lost its last chance. The tears are a different loss: not the loss of a person necessarily but the loss of an opportunity, the final loss of a relationship. People with deep and loving commitments often feel immense loss but not regret. They know the relationship was loving and that whatever issues they had between themselves were manageable, not obstacles to their love and friendship. But when the relationship between parent and child was a constant source of friction or that between a husband and wife was filled with acrimony, the mourning is often not over the death of the person but the death of possibility. When you watch a family go fully into the tunnel of grief, you know that they will come out the other end, but they don't always know. They believe that sadness is the new normal, that every day will be overcast, that laughter is reserved for others but not for them. And then the cocoon that held them for so long in the stillness of grief breaks, and they look back sentimentally on a happier ending and may even be able to imagine one for themselves, not because they erase the pain or block it from memory but because the distance gives them something that the immediacy of anguish cannot: perspective.

Faye had been dying for years. And while we are all moving toward death, Faye moved, in the last five weeks of her life, much faster than anyone else I knew. Faye had cancer that had begun in her breast and then metastasized into something more insidious, infecting her bones and her brain and riddling through her so that it impacted her eyesight and her ability to stand up straight. Then it attacked her voice; the same unwanted guest that took over her life would soon take her life altogether. Her skin became jaundiced because her kidneys no longer worked. In addition to her yellowing skin, she was bruised all over; the black and blue marks had a reddish undertone. The automatic morphine drip diminished her pain but amplified the anguish of her family and friends; she was slowly losing coherence.

Intellectually, I knew we were losing Faye before she died. But when the hospice workers arrived at the house, I suddenly felt it was imminent, a matter of days, maybe weeks at most. She lay in bed most days, able to respond with only a word or two. As Mark, her devoted husband, said, "When we brought her home five weeks ago, she could have a whole conversation. Four weeks ago she spoke in a few sentences. Three weeks ago she could only respond with a sentence.

Two weeks ago, she had only a few words. In the last week, she didn't say anything." The evolution of silence. Death has a painful way of usurping language. Mark had a consolation prize: "The last thing she said to me a few days ago was 'I love you.' She used to hold my hand. But yesterday, her hands were just soft and open, as if they could hold nothing anymore. And then I knew it would be soon."

Who are you if you are merely a physical shell? I asked myself that dozens of times during Faye's five long weeks of descent into death. Even the very last day of her life, when I went to visit her in the morning, I heard the idiosyncratic Chicago lilt in her cough and knew it was still Faye. But I was holding on to the scraps of selfhood, the small leftovers that were soon to disappear. I was never sure exactly what she understood of our conversations, but I know they were not one-sided, not until the very last days.

Watching Faye's transition in those five weeks made me aware of an important trajectory shared with me by my friend and colleague Greg, a rabbi who escorts people through this process too often. "Between sickness and death is the sacred transition of the dying process." When you are sick, you have to put all of your energies into fighting sickness. When you are dying, you have to resign yourself to an end and repair what you can and give your last gifts and words to others. There is space in between fighting and resignation. That space represents the process of dying; it is the one that most of us ignore. It is the one that we can sanctify. It may just be the most important time in our lives.

Faye and I got to know each other through our daughters, who were the new kids in sixth grade and immediately bonded with each other. They are in college together now. Faye developed breast cancer a year after we met, when Samantha was only thirteen and her brother was nine. She had wonderful care at Johns Hopkins, one of the best hospitals in the world, and went into remission for four years. As she once said, "They told me if I hit five years I would be good. But I didn't make it to then." She battled cancer hard with every ounce of her limited strength. She had a core of belief in God that sustained her, and when her oncologist finally said that he was unwilling to subject her to more pain through experimental treatment, she didn't resign herself to an end she didn't want. "It's all in God's hands." I heard her say that dozens of times.

We discussed our kids and our expectations and disappointments, but I felt a wave of privilege when we spoke because, through some act of grace, I would continue to have these conversations. Faye would not. I did not feel more deserving. Just luckier for now.

Grieving when death comes from illness begins long before the final end. We mourn the people who become shadows of themselves. When a friend began dating after the death of his beloved wife to cancer, someone cornered him, surprised. "But Andrea just died a few months ago."

"To me," he whispered, "the Andrea I fell in love with died four years ago."

Happy endings must be both about the dying managing death better and the living managing the death of those we love better.

Mark slept on the floral couch beside Faye's hospital bed in the family room. He had not slept more than three to four hours a night in the last weeks of Faye's life. He wanted to hold on to the little pieces left of Faye, no matter how small. "I never wished death upon her, even when I knew she wasn't herself and that everything was getting harder and harder. I never believed it would be better for her to die than to live. Doctors gave us predictions of how much time we had left together, and I believed them. Faye never did."

Faye knew about illness close up. Her father sold shoes and was the breadwinner of the family, but that stopped when he got leukemia. An only child, she dropped out of a carefree schoolgirl life as an adolescent to care for her dying father. Faye spent ten years as his caretaker and the family anchor. Her mother didn't drive, so when Faye got her license, she chauffeured her dad around to doctors' appointments and pharmacies, running the errands of the dying. She was no stranger to illness or death. When she and Mark received her diagnosis, Faye turned to her husband and said, "I feel sorry for you."

"Sorry for me?" Mark replied. But Faye understood all too well the price of illness on the caretakers. Years fighting cancer gave her a kind of mental callousness about death, but for Mark the bruise of it all was still tender.

On the desk once used for work was the detritus of illness, the pills and boxes of face masks and plastic gloves, the creams and ointments and adult diapers, a hideous display of the dependencies and indignities of cancer. Just opposite the bed was a collection of books on the shelves; some had the normal titles of books appropriate for a family of four. And then on a few shelves titles snuck in alluding to the vast, hovering plague that had taken over the house. *How to Fight Cancer and Win* stared at me until I turned its spine inward, accusing the book as I flipped it of selling false optimism. Where was *How to Fight Cancer and Lose?* That's what I really needed to read for guidance. Soon, all the books and medicine and signs of sickness would be moved out, as if Faye never occupied this space, almost like a hotel room that returns to its anonymity when all the stuff of an occupant's life is removed.

There were things Faye wanted to finish before she died. She had a children's book she was writing, about a little girl who wanted to make wigs for a living. No doubt this idea came to her when she began losing her own hair from the chemotherapy. Mark made sure she dictated the end, when the little girl finally meets a wigmaker and sees how wigs are cut. When she told me to read it, my first thought was: *Good, another thing she wanted to finish checked off the list.* Faye was a teacher for most of her adult life, but she enjoyed writing, and knowing that her written words would be collected and published pleased her.

Faye also wanted to travel down memory lane with Mark and review the life they had together. Mark decided to hang pictures that had accumulated over the years but had never been displayed. "We had our picture taken at Sears or Penney's every six months, but they all just sat in boxes. Now all of a sudden every picture seems important." Mark spent the better part of a week hanging the family pictures in the upstairs hallway, thinking that Faye would see them on the way upstairs. But only a few days later, she could no longer be moved upstairs.

She also wanted to leave goodbye videos for her two children and one for Mark, which they taped when she was taken back to the hospital during her hospice treatment. I imagined Mark zooming in on Faye's sallow face as she left her remarks for him to treasure once she was gone. Mark told me on one visit that they had recorded a message for the yet-unconceived grandchildren. Another painful act but an important piece of unfinished business that was completed.

Saying goodbye to Faye seemed to take too long. I would avoid the agonizing sense of despair and waiting by looking for things to do as she lay still in the bed. Faye was an avid reader of fantasy novels, and as her eyes began to fail, she was unable to get to the end of *Brisingr*, the third book in a Christopher Paolini fantasy series and more than 700 pages long. She stopped in the mid-600s. She was frustrated that she hadn't finished it before the growth in her brain began to affect her eyesight, leaving her cross-eyed at times and making reading an immense challenge.

I read to her. Faye wore a navy fisherman's hat, and you could see the light fuzz of her rounded head at the periphery of the hat. She closed her eyes and concentrated on the words, clearly deriving pleasure in the listening. *Brisingr* has a wide cast of characters, elves and winged-bird creatures and dragon types, with complex Scandinavian names. For the life of me, as I read, I had no idea what was going on. But Faye did. I thought I could cheat the angel of death because he clearly would not bother someone midchapter. A friend who volunteers in a library told me that she had made a deal with God: God could not take her life until she had finished all the books in her personal library. "That's why I keep buying more books," she told me offhandedly, as if that were the most compelling and obvious reason to buy books rather than check them out of the library in which she herself worked.

What difference would it make if Faye stopped at page 698 instead of 748, our reading destination? She was not going to get to volume four, which, as of our reading, was not yet written. I didn't know how to answer that question, except to say that we must get to 748.

We advanced a few sentences: "Later on—no matter how careful we are, if we live long enough, eventually one of us will die. It is not a happy thought, but it is the truth. Such is the way of the world." And then: "Shifting his stance, Oromis said, 'I cannot pretend that I regard this with favor, but the purpose of life is not to do what we want but what needs to be done. This is what fate demands of us.'" *Fate demands something of us*: I thought of this line again and again.

What needs to be done?

What needs to be done?

Finally we arrived at the last page. On page 749, we read together: "Here ends the third book of the Inheritance Cycle. The story will continue and conclude in book four." I let out a sigh. We got there.

So what?

•   •   •

I asked Mark if he had granted Faye permission to die. Maybe she was holding on because she believed people needed her. "No. I haven't. We just never talked to each other that way." He didn't want to give her permission to die, only permission to live.

"All I want is to live to see both my children married and grand-children. Well, even if I can't see all my grandchildren that would be all right . . . just a few would be good." That is all Faye asked of God. And she imagined that perhaps it was too much to ask. Faye studied religious texts and prayed fervently every day, "in the hope that God would grant me my wish to be a *bubbie*." She spoke to God every day. But God did not grant her this simple wish that so many others are blessed to have. I felt selfish and hopeless talking to her, as if I should not have what she could not have. I wanted to give her the impossible.

Faye had many people who prayed for her recovery, myself in-cluded. It was important to her that we continue to pray to the very end. Praying for those who are sick is an ancient biblical tradition, dating back to Moses in the twelfth chapter of Numbers, where he prayed for his sister Miriam: "Please, God, heal her." These four sim-ple words of compassion and urgency became the basis of a tradition of praying for others. Praying on someone else's behalf helps us un-derstand their pain and contribute to their healing. There have been many medical studies on the effects of intercessory prayer; even when people are praying for a total stranger, there seem to be some health benefits when the patient believes he or she is the subject of prayer.[2]

I did not embark on this practice myself until I was quite sick. My illness was not life-threatening, but I had missed a few weeks of work and felt anger that my body had let me down and let down my kids, who needed more strength and energy from me than I had. I returned to the classroom to teach, and our study group asked me to stand as they formed a prayer circle around me. They made a blessing of thanks that I had reached the day when I could come back to teach them. I was so stunned by it that my eyes welled, and I realized how loved I felt in those few minutes of fellowship. I was not alone, even though illness can be profoundly isolating. From then on I began to pray daily for those who are sick and for many who are dying. Prayer matters to them, and I feel humbled and grateful when I pray for others, some of whom I will never meet.

But I could not grant Faye's last wish. Prayer can only go so far. I wanted to help her think about her last days and what she wanted to say and how to proceed into the last passage and finality with the fortitude that she had in abundance. She seemed ready, and I thought of something Mary Callanan said in *Final Journeys*: "By the time they are close to dying, they usually have reached an emotional state of acceptance and actually *want* to go forward into whatever awaits them."[3] I felt that time was upon us.

Once when Faye had gone out of hospice care and back into the hospital for intense pain management, I walked in when she was reading a love poem she wrote to Mark when they were dating. They met on a plane in 1982 traveling from Miami to Chicago. Mark was returning from a visit with his parents. Ironically, Faye was coming back from an unsuccessful singles' weekend that suddenly looked like it might have a very successful end. They were engaged two months later. Faye was smiling in the hospital while Mark videotaped her reading the words of the love poem and reliving the memory of that time in their lives together. I winced when I imagined him playing this after Faye was gone, maybe in the middle of the night when the bedroom is half empty and he has trouble sleeping; Larkin's words haunt again: "But I have watched all night / The fire grow silent." When she came back from the hospital, he taped her poem to the wall close to her bed. I thought of the ancient verse from the Song of Songs, "Let me be a seal upon your heart, like the seal upon your hand, for love is as fierce as death."[4]

Fierceness describes certain kinds of love. Love can feel light and soft or hazy and fuzzy. But that's not what I was watching. I was watching an urgent, sharp, anguished love, and it was fierce. And like the biblical verse, it seemed that Mark was trying to seal every last moment with Faye.

In the ancient world, people regularly marked their bodies with the modern-day equivalent of tattoos to mourn their dead. They would permanently seal a mark in their flesh, as if to make a statement with their very bodies that all cannot be the same with the onset of grief. We are permanently marked by loss. It cannot be other than this. In the ancient Middle East it was common when in mourning to gash the flesh and remove the hair, believing that these actions would have an effect on the ghost of the dead person, either as an offering to strengthen the ghost in the netherworld or to make the ghost less jealous of the living. If the mourners are physically and emotionally torn apart, then perhaps being alive is not so enviable. Others interpret the gashing and hair tearing as signs of guilt. In sixth-century Athens, mourners were forbidden to tear at themselves to evoke pity, and women in fifth-century Rome were not allowed to lacerate their cheeks.[5] Deuteronomy specifically forbids this practice: "You are the children of the Lord your God. You shall not gash yourselves or shave the front of your heads because of the dead."[6] The beginning of the verse stresses that we are all God's children, meaning that we all have self-worth since we are created in the divine image, and the loss of someone we love should hurt us but not paralyze us or lead to despair. It is for this reason that Jews are forbidden by the Torah to tattoo themselves.

We've all seen the residual ink of post-girlfriend tattoos. They are near impossible to remove. You may no longer have her in your life, but you have some memory of her on your skin, even if you've been through laser removal. No one person should have that impact on anyone. The prohibition against tattoos in Jewish law centers on not making anyone in our lives so significant that it marks us for life. One eighteenth-century commentary on the verse in Deuteronomy follows this approach to grief: "No personality may chain us so closely to it, allow us to be so absorbed into it, as having no longer any value, as would be what the permanent sign of cut or baldness on our body is meant to express."[7] This Bible interpreter stresses "our own self-valuation even against our nearest and dearest."[8] Grief is mandatory. Paralysis is prohibited.

During each of my visits, Mark entered the room and asked Faye if she needed anything, then kissed her forehead or lightly brushed her cheek with his hand. In these small gestures of togetherness, I saw a couple preserving the glue that brought them together, keeping the love alive before it all unraveled. In his eulogy, Mark mentioned that he and Faye were married for twenty-nine years, and in that time she went through twenty-two operations. Mark was by her side throughout. The toll on the caregiver in such situations is immense. Maggie Callanan regrets how few caregivers get the help they need because they suffer the situation alone, believing that they can handle the trouble or that it is a test of the relationship to go it alone: "All too often I have seen two ambulances arrive at the house of a patient—one for the patient and one for the caregiver." Callanan began to tell patients and their families: "I only allow one patient per address."[9]

For three and a half years, Mark accompanied Faye to every

chemotherapy and radiation treatment. He was with her virtually all day and all night every day for her last five weeks of life. As Mark tells it, "In the very end, when she drank juice from an eyedropper or ate a bit of pudding from a spoon, and choked while she spoke, we repeated 'I love you' over and over and then over again." I know those words well because I would always say "I love you" to Faye when I left and she'd repeat it back to me each time until she could no longer speak. The last time we had a conversation, I told her that she looked beautiful. There was something very radiant about her deep blue eyes, especially without hair. The very last thing she said to me was, "By the way, you're beautiful too."

Faye saw Mark's intense commitment and how things had changed. "We have a lot of romance now. We never used to have time for romance, but now we do. Last week we had a whole day to ourselves in the hospital." Faye shared this new and welcome dimension of their last weeks together. It was not to last.

Faye died on a Saturday night. Against all odds, she lived through another Passover and another Sabbath, two dates of great importance on the Jewish calendar. My daughter called to tell me. It was ten forty-five. I had seen Faye that morning. There was a sharp increase in her heart rate, and she was no longer responsive to conversation. Her eyes remained closed for more than two days. She let out small, animal-like noises every once in a while. After the Sabbath, Mark went to his study to check e-mails and came up to find her not breathing. Soon, half a dozen people were in different parts of the house, making arrangements for the burial, speaking to Mark, hugging Samantha. Their son was stoic and quiet. We came over after midnight to share in the bedlam and confusion.

The night she passed away, while we waited for the funeral

personnel to remove the body, Faye's outline under the sheets suddenly seemed so small. I almost thought they had already taken her and just left the covers on the bed. I removed the cloth over her face to say goodbye. Samantha didn't want to see her mother like that. She wanted to hold on to the living mother she recognized, not the mother who sank into the ether of sickness and finally surrendered. Sitting on the couch opposite a wedding picture of him and Faye, Mark told us quietly that he would never hold on to the images of what Faye looked like now. Pointing to the framed photo, he said, "That's who I will always remember." His bride.

We stayed with Mark and his children until the funeral home staff removed Faye's body. It was about one thirty in the morning, but there was no real sense of time in the room. When they moved the body out of the house, there was another emotional tremor for the family. It was all part of the fits and starts of mourning, the moments of calm and clarity counterpointed by sudden gasps of shock.

Mark prepared his remarks for the funeral. He had spoken to me about them weeks earlier but only handed me a copy the morning that Faye died. I committed not to read Mark's eulogy before Faye died, irrationally believing that reading the notes prematurely would bring about her death. I am not superstitious. At least most of the time.

In Jewish tradition, the first day of mourning is called *aninut,* a state of suspension from normal activities. Because the mourner in the first shock of death has difficulty focusing and may be struggling with profound religious questions, he or she is exempted from prayer and other Jewish ritual activities to immerse in the needs of the dead and to allow time for confronting raw pain before moving on to the next stage of mourning. At the house with Mark and his children the night Faye died, I understood this suspension. Everything was surreal. Every phone call strange. Every question that had to be answered felt wrong, like a betrayal. One of the great Jewish philosophers of the twentieth century, Rabbi Joseph Soloveitchik, describes this first stage of mourning as "the spontaneous human reaction to death":

> It is an outcry, a shout, or a howl of grisly horrors and disgust. Man responds to his defeat at the hands of death with total resignation and with an all-consuming masochistic, self-devastating black despair. Beaten by the fiend, his prayers rejected, enveloped by a hideous darkness, forsaken and lonely, man begins to question his own human singular reality.[10]

The mourner's most profound crises are allowed, indeed, encouraged to surface at this stage. It is perfectly normal to question not only the death of the beloved but also all death, including one's own. It is unavoidable. Death throws mourners into immense existential strife.

Nothing is yet scripted; initially, it is the mourner who determines the emotional response to the loss. This gives way during the funeral and burial to a highly orchestrated set of rituals that carry the mourner from shock to cognitive acceptance, from the incapacity to speak to the ability to remember the life through a loving narrative epitomized by eulogies and the stories told at the *shiva*, which re-creates the portrait of the deceased with friends and community. A very private friend who had a brother in public life had hundreds of mourners in her home the week after she lost her mother. I asked her if she found all the attention difficult, given her personality. "On the contrary," she said, as she sat on a low stool in her parents' living room. "Each person has brought me another piece of my mother." The howl at the onset of loss is gradually replaced with the wonder of story. In the words of Rabbi Soloveitchik, the mourner must undertake a heroic task: "to start picking up the debris of his own shattered personality and reestablish himself as man, restoring lost glory, dignity, and uniqueness."[11]

Jews have extensive and intricate mourning rituals. The Jewish mourner speaks first when being visited. He or she is responsible for the conversation—or for the silence. Grief is highly subjective; consequently, we hand over that subjectivity to the mourner to determine the atmosphere in which to mourn. Nevertheless, one is regarded as cruel if he or she cannot mourn the loss of a loved one. Death should make us introspective and open to repentance as we check our own deeds. But Jewish law does not only direct itself to those who refuse to mourn. It also chastises those who overly mourn:

> One should not grieve too much for the dead, and whosoever grieves excessively is actually grieving for someone else. The Torah sets limits for each step of grieving and we may add to them: three for weeping, seven for lamenting, and 30 for refraining from wearing clean clothes and cutting hair—*and no more.*[12]

The law is describing a progression of both mourning and emerging from mourning. During the initial seven-day mourning period, the *shiva*, the synagogue is effectively brought into the home: the *minyan*, a quorum required for certain rites, and prayerbooks are moved to allow the mourner to say *Kaddish,* the prayer for the dead, at home. At the end of *shiva*, the mourner walks around the block to symbolize that he or she has come out of the bubble of weeping and is ready, even in a fragile and shaky state, to re-enter the community of the living. Not being able to do so is regarded as a spiritual blemish on the mourner.

• • •

Faye's funeral was on Holocaust Remembrance Day, and the day after news broke that Osama bin Laden was dead. Mourning for the victims of genocide took place next to a death that was anticipated, even celebrated, around the United States. Faye's death did not make the news smaller. It just magnified the loss of so many people to the Holocaust and to World War II and 9/11 because each family is a universe, each story its own tragedy.

It was a beautiful spring day, too sunny to lose a wife and a mother. Too sunny to lose a friend. Hundreds of people filed into the synagogue. I helped Samantha tear the garment close to her skin, a Jewish ritual representing the breaking of a heart, right before the family entered the social hall where the eulogies were to be given. I had helped Diane tear her garment when Alyssa died and watched her sink into my arms. She said she could feel her heart rip.

Often you find that the people who speak at a funeral offer differing portraits of the person being eulogized; a collective, layered picture begins to emerge. Every once in a while you find a familiar strain or repeated pattern in every eulogy, indicating the strength of a person's character. A former student once told me that she lost a friend, and every one of the seven people who spoke at the service said that the young woman never said a bad word about anyone. What a startling end and tribute.

At Faye's funeral, every single speech highlighted her tenacity, her strength in the face of illness and her unshakable faith. The woman who spoke right before me said many of the things that I had on the paper I was holding. I was in no state to change a word, and then I realized that I didn't have to change anything. This was Faye. This is who she was to me. If she was the same thing to others then so be it. Maybe it will have some staying power with those listening. Maybe her image will stay longer with me. My voice was shaky. I had to stop twice: once when I said that Mark's devotion gave meaning to the expression "in sickness and in health," and a second time when I shuddered at the fact that her deepest wish, to be a grandmother, would never be realized and that, in the last weeks, she pulled back her request, not asking God to see all of her grandchildren but only a few. My hands twitched the whole while. There was the surreal sense that this wasn't really happening, combined with the inevitability that it was really happening. This is all there ever really is in the construct of a human being. Birth. Death. I held the speech so tightly that my nails dug into my palms and then I sat down.

Gasps and sighs limned the audience, the background music to so many funerals. Mark heaved with tears several times, as if to say, *I can't believe today is the day I am burying my wife.* It was Mark's sixtieth birthday; Samantha's twentieth birthday was the day before. Every subsequent birthday would, no doubt, carry with it the weight of this awful day.

In Jewish custom, all rituals involving death are called *hesed shel emet*, "the loving-kindness of truth." Acts of kindness, *hesed*, are regarded as the basic transactional currency of a meaningful life in community. Often good deeds are done with a utilitarian mindset, the *quid pro quo* of goodness, so to speak. Kindnesses done for the dead are regarded with greater significance, since they cannot be reciprocated by the recipients. One such ritual is accompanying the body some distance to its next journey. Upon completion of the eulogies, pallbearers remove the casket and place it in a hearse. The community walks behind them, and the vehicle that takes the body to the cemetery drives slowly for a few dozen feet so the community

can symbolically continue the journey and offer a dignified show of strength and communion as a send-off.

Faye's casket and the blue velvet mantle that covered it was eased from the pallbearers' hold and pushed into the back of a van rather than a hearse. The casket was not going to a cemetery. It was going to the airport. We moved from the stark, air-conditioned hall into the bright sunlight of a midmorning spring day. My daughter held Samantha's hand as she walked the slow walk of loss. The van drove through the parking lot to the road's first intersection. Mark heaved into his son's shoulder and shuffled ahead. We got to the stop sign, and again Mark cried out. The van picked up speed on the way to the airport and, ultimately, the finality of burial. I stood watching the van until it turned the corner, out of sight. Faye was gone.

The family stood in the street, in the stillness of an impossible thought: a wife and mother was gone. Gone. They waited for their transportation to the airport. As I turned to go home, blinking in the sunlight, I thought of the words of W. B. Yeats:

> *Though leaves are many, the root is one;*
> *Through all the lying days of my youth,*
> *I swayed my leaves and flowers in the sun;*
> *Now I may wither into the truth.*

It took me days to leave the funeral.

Faye was buried in Israel about twenty minutes outside of Jerusalem in a peaceful, wooded cemetery. It was her last wish. Bleary-eyed, the family left the funeral for the airport and spent a dizzying thirty-six hours in Israel, interrupted the morning after the burial when

Samantha couldn't find her passport, forcing them to miss their flight home and take another flight. It's not hard to see how this might happen in the daze of mourning, but it felt like another hiccup in the tragic narrative of Faye's end. I went with a friend to prepare the house for the *shiva*. The family sits on low chairs and are supposed to focus only on the one lost. They do not bathe or change clothing for the duration of the week except in preparation for the Sabbath, when the *shiva* is temporarily suspended.

The hospice bed and all the medical equipment had to be removed. I packed manila folder after manila folder of X-rays into a cardboard box and put them in the basement. We opened the windows and tried to get the humidity of death that lingered so potently for weeks out of the house. We put things away; the cleaning was both compassionate and invasive. We were sorting through the stuff of sickness, the film of cancer that touched inanimate objects everywhere. Each object seemed to hold up a different aspect of Faye. For me, the hardest was the wedding photograph in the living room. Faye had wanted them both to wear white. She looked so young, and Mark wore the kind of white polyester tuxedo that he later explained came with the hotel wedding package in Chicago. The whiteness of it is filled with so much innocence and expectation.

Mark confided in me that he wanted just one more day with Faye. What is one more day? I thought. A friend returning from the funeral of an elderly man who was "supposed" to have died several months earlier said that in one of the eulogies a family member got up and offered the doctor's sour predictions for public scrutiny. In the short span of months beyond the death date that this man was given, he managed to be part of the weddings of two of his grandchildren and alive for the births of five great-grandchildren. One more day is still one more day.

• • •

A contemporary scholar of religion, Rabbi Irving Greenberg, speaks about a final cutoff from intimate personal experience. His son J.J. was killed biking at age thirty-six when a van ran a light. His parents saw him twenty-four hours earlier but then never again. When Greenberg describes the rip that takes someone out of the fabric of a life, he and his family have the scars to prove it. I wrote a condolence letter to the family when J.J. died, and all I could say was "There are no words." It felt wholly inadequate to say it and then mail it, but I did anyway. Irving's wife, Blu, wrote back:

"Yes. There are no words."

At the moment I read the card, it seemed the most honest exchange of grief that ever took place.

This prompts the irrational but unshakable belief that nothing else can or should continue when life draws to an end. There can never be another sunny day; every laugh is a slap. The death fog, the haziness of grief that encases the newly bereaved, often sends out a grim message to others: I will never smile again. I can never really walk, talk, *be* again in the wake of this loss.

Research today tells us that not all love lost is the same. Men and women experience grieving differently.[13] One man who lost his wife of fifty-three years wouldn't go to a bereavement support group because it was all women. "I just didn't think women would relate to my pain. . . . And, frankly, I come from a generation that feels uncomfortable exposing our sadness and vulnerability to the opposite sex."[14] His anxieties are mirrored in what we know today about widowers having more psychological and physical signs of illness and depression after their loss than do women. According to Michael Caserta, chairman of the Center for Healthy Aging at the University of Utah: "While women who lose their husbands often speak of feeling abandoned or deserted, widowers tend to experience the loss as one of dismemberment, as if they had lost something that kept them organized and whole."[15] This sense of dismemberment is aggravated by emotional expectations that men stay strong and keep their feelings tucked deep inside. As a result, a grief specialist who works with men says that she never asks men how they are feeling but rather asks them what they are doing, a question that generally surfaces their despair gently rather than head-on.

One widower who couldn't keep his thoughts to himself has brought solace to thousands of men *and* women in the throes of anguish. C. S. Lewis captured his pain in great detail in the journal he kept after his wife, Helen Joy Davidman, died. It was later published as A *Grief Observed*. Lewis met Davidman under very unusual circumstances. Lewis was a British intellectual giant who, from 1954 until 1963, held a literature chair at Cambridge University and was an articulate defender of Christianity. Davidman, an American writer, communist and intellectual, was a married woman, an atheist daughter of two Jewish parents. Davidman was interested in Lewis's writings on religion and began a robust correspondence with him that ended in her conversion to Christianity.

When Davidman's own marriage ended in divorce, she and her two sons moved to the same town as Lewis outside Oxford, ostensibly to deepen their friendship and intellectual companionship. They had a civil union to facilitate her stay in the United Kingdom, but the relationship remained platonic until she developed bone cancer in 1956. Only then did this confirmed bachelor decide to marry her, knowing that her life was marked and that, according to the Church of England, which did not sanction divorce, this marriage was not religiously acceptable. A friend performed the ceremony at her hospital bed.

They had only four brief years to spend together as a wedded couple, but Lewis observed that this time made an indelible impression on his sense of self: "The most precious gift that marriage gave me was this constant impact of something very close and intimate yet all the time unmistakably other, resistant—in a word, real."[16]

Otherness, that vaguely difficult quality that attracts and repels us, is not something we always assume we'll miss, but it is the very otherness of someone close to us that stands out most after loss. We grasp for that which is unlike us. Rabbi Greenberg writes beautifully of the connection between love and death that attenuates the power of love precisely because of its fragility and otherness:

> In its truest form, love wants to always be with the Other; the lover is filled with joy and well being when helping and sharing with the Other. Love makes one want to be with the beloved forever, in life, in vital shared experience, in joint mission. But here love meets the cruelest foe, death. Death is the enemy of love. It robs the loved one of his/her value, equality and uniqueness. Death snatches the irreplaceable one, the one I have become so attached to, the one so inextricably bound up in the web of my existence—and rips that one out of the fabric of my life. The wound is raw and hard to heal. Oh, for just one more time to hear the gentle voice, one more embrace and kiss, one more smile, one more shared kindness, laughter, joy, one more task done together to fulfillment. But it is not possible. The cutoff is final. The yearned-for moment is denied.[17]

One more time. One more time. Just to speak, to kiss, to embrace that person one more time. But it would not be enough. One more time would soon ease into one time after that. How could it not?

During the weeks following Davidman's death, Lewis kept a journal in which he refers to Joy merely as "H." He decided to publish his early ruminations on loss if it would help others confront the specter of a life partner dying. He used whatever notebooks lay about the house but refused to buy anything else to write on, believing that his morbid musings should come to an end by the time he ran out of paper. He wrote for a modicum of comfort, but even that was strained: "Part of every misery is, so to speak, the misery's shadow or reflection: the fact that you don't merely suffer but have to keep on thinking about the fact that you suffer. I not only live each endless day in grief, but live each day thinking about living each day in grief."[18]

His mind was preoccupied, his everyday life flat and undifferentiated. He knew that others looked at him with pity and even embarrassment. When he passed a happily married couple, he was aware that they looked at him with sadness, knowing that he represented what would one day befall them: ultimate separation. Some in Lewis's social circle shunned him when he married Davidman. He believed that his stepson, a teenager at the time, also felt embarrassment around him, uncomfortable with the tragic cloud that trailed Lewis, awkward about the love that had downed this rational thinker. Douglas Gresham, the stepson mentioned, wrote an introduction to A Grief Observed as an adult and believes that Lewis mistook Gresham's own grief for embarrassment. He was closed about his mother's death, mimicking the appropriate cultural response he assumed was his responsibility as a fourteen-year-old British preparatory school student. But had Lewis really spoken to him of his mother, he would have, he confessed, wept uncontrollably. Gresham writes that it took him thirty years to cry without feeling ashamed.

Lewis worked hard to capture his emotional landscape; he was visiting a place wholly foreign to him, and, like a travel writer, he immersed himself in the place's intensity. Grief to him felt like fear or, oddly, like suspense:

Or like waiting; just hanging about waiting for something to happen. It gives life a permanently provisional feeling. It doesn't seem worth starting anything. I can't settle down. I yawn, I fidget, I smoke too much. Up till this I always had too little time. Now there is nothing but time. Almost pure time, empty successiveness.[19]

Lewis struggled to find the language to describe the weeks and months after Davidman's death. Everyday tasks like shaving seemed burdensome and pointless. Rough or smooth, what did it matter? To whom did it matter anymore? Lewis worried that his self-pity made him too self-absorbed. He thought not of H. but of himself. And when he finally emerged ever slightly from his bath of grief, Lewis experienced shame at saying that he felt better, believing that he was under an obligation to foment his unhappiness, otherwise he was betraying his lover. We want, he says, to "prove to ourselves that we are lovers on a grand scale, tragic heroes,"[20] not just commoners who accept fate and move on, however difficult. We don't want grief, but we don't *not* want it. Grieving means that we are still attached, still powerfully connected to the deceased.

Richard Neuhaus, a Christian theologian, describes the self-absorption of grief in a slightly different way. He walked in the world of grief in a totally different mindset than everyone else, a state of disbelief:

As much as I was grateful for all the calls and letters, I harbored a secret resentment. These friends who said they were thinking about me and praying for me all the time, I knew they also went shopping and visited their children and tended to their businesses, and there were long times when they were not thinking about me at all. More important, they were forgetting the primordial, overwhelming, indomitable fact: we are dying![21]

Death becomes so tangible, so close, that it touches everything, soils everything, spoils everything. Like frost, it covers everything in a chilling membrane; everything that is exposed is touched by it. The person wrapped up in death, whether in mourning for a loved one or facing one's own death, cannot imagine any mundane task eclipsing the prominence of death, the way that it sucks all the air out of the room. It dominates all thoughts. That small exclamation mark Neuhaus uses—we are dying!—says so much about the distance between someone confronting mortality and someone who is not.

C. S. Lewis is known as a staunch apologist for Christianity; it was strange, therefore, to read about the turn that religion took in his mind when Davidman died. He knew he would not be the same. He just didn't know how. Religion at a time of grief is supposed to be a source of comfort. Instead, it became part of the problem:

> The old life, the jokes, the drinks, the arguments, the lovemaking, the tiny heartbreaking commonplace. On any view whatever, to say "H. is dead," is to say "All that is gone." It is part of the past. And the past is the past and that is what time means, and time itself is one more name for death, and Heaven itself is a state where "the former things have passed away." Talk to me about truth of religion and I'll listen gladly. Talk to me about the duty of religion and I'll listen submissively. But don't come talking to me about the consolations of religion or I shall suspect that you don't understand.[22]

Religion was not a soft pillow for Lewis.

Ultimately, it seems that humility in the face of death, and only humility, is a tenable response. We don't know what or how we will feel. We ask not to be judged. We do not know with any certainty what will bring solace. Presumed sources of consolation are often disappointments. In grief, we abide in the silence between words.

• • •

In the months that followed Faye's death, I thought often about the dignity of silence. I also kept returning to a paragraph from Mark's eulogy that explained so much about grief and so much about love:

> We knew that our love extended beyond faith—we remained at different levels of observance and spirituality; beyond family—we wanted to be with each other more than we even wanted to be with the kids; and beyond friends, we cherished the time when no one was around. However, in all our long goodbyes, we never did figure out why we loved each other so very much. . . . Our love was a labyrinth of choices, practices, and emotions that is difficult to put into words.

They were so different, Mark and Faye. And those differences ultimately mattered a great deal and not at all. They mattered because it was the contrast that made each of them stand out in relation to the other. The capacity to note those differences and appreciate them made the grieving over Faye much richer and more intense. It didn't matter because the love they had transcended those differences. They didn't have to figure out love. It just existed. It was the labyrinth of choices that had no set language of reason. And the grieving over the loss of a love that held so much mystery is bound to be deeper and more complex. Despite the language that could not be found, they had used their last weeks to confront all that was necessary. In Mark's words, "All that could be said about our lives together was said."

Managing grief suddenly seemed possible to me in ways that it had not before Faye died. Mark showed me the color of love. In the totality of his grief, he showed me a happier ending because grief was an extension of his love, its natural shadow. Happier endings are not about unadulterated joy at the prospect of death. They imply death with a rich texture of meaning and substance, the process of achieving closeness and the attempt at emptying oneself in the intake of another. The grief is the underside of intimacy. It is the profile of darkness on the sidewalk that is the same shape as the person but slightly more amplified. Faye was the shadow now and not the person. She was both larger as a shadow and more ephemeral. You saw her and then did not. She appears, but only in the most diaphanous of ways. You cannot catch a shadow. But you can see a shadow.

I spoke with many grieving people who believe that their loved one appears to them in the shape of an animal, especially a bird. There are late-night visitations or appearances where they are least expected. Mourners turn a corner and a wind catches them too abruptly. An item on a desk is suddenly not where it was left. Who moved it? This is not superstition speaking. It is the voice of a disrupted rhythm that cannot right itself. It is the shadow speaking, the imprint of a voice or an expression that repeats itself, again and again, whispering to us, making decisions with us, telling us what to do. It is the sudden warmth that envelops us in a time of joy. It is the chill that we cannot shake.

It is the way that people leave us and never really leave us.

## Chapter Ten

# Using Death to Change Your Life

Alyssa's death was real, so was Dennis's death. And Faye's. The woman I ritually bathed was dead too. But over time, I learned that my search for the better death involved not only the concrete death of individuals but the theoretical deaths of us all. If death is a fact of existence, then how can the *idea* of death, not only the act of dying, change our lives?

Mary Oliver, the Pulitzer Prize–winning American poet, captured death's teachings with a snatch of meaning in her poem "When Death Comes." She describes death's arrival as an iceberg between the shoulder blades, that which steals the bright coins from a purse. Eternity in her poem becomes another possibility for using death to change a life:

*When it's over, I want to say: all my life*
*I was a bride married to amazement.*
*I was a bridegroom, taking the world into my arms.*
*When it's over, I don't want to wonder*
*if I have made of my life something particular, and real.*
*I don't want to find myself sighing and frightened,*
*or full of argument.*
*I don't want to end up simply having visited this world.*

"Married to amazement": a remarkable expression, really. That kind of marriage is an achievement that perhaps only death can force. Without death, we might never take the world fully into our arms. We might never achieve wisdom. We would just wait another day. "I can be kind tomorrow. I can be smart tomorrow." We will have visited the world but never really lived in it. Alternatively, we can adopt Oliver's amazement about life that helps manage the fear of dying: "I want to step through the door full of curiosity, wondering; what is it going to be like, that cottage of darkness?"

We can turn to ancient literature to enter that cottage of darkness and see if it helps us use death to live life better. When I'm in that cottage, I find myself turning to the book of Job. Job, the suffering man of the Bible who had insufferable friends, understood that although death and trouble beset him, his tragic experiences contributed to greater knowledge. When I teach Job, I've often asked my adult students to pair themselves up and open to any chapter in the book arbitrarily, read the entire chapter with each other and discuss its approach to suffering with each other. I generally cannot task people with opening to any chapter of the Bible and finding meaning there because the awkward translations and density of the ancient text are difficult. But I am confident that whatever chapter they turn to in Job will yield profound insights, and so far it's worked. Job's lyricism about the human condition often moves people to tears as they share its verses out loud, reviewing darker moments in their lives as Job articulates their own anguish: "I am disgusted with life. I will give reign to my complaint, speak in the bitterness of my soul. I say to God, 'Do not condemn me; let me know what You charge me with'" (10:1–2).

Job, as the old legend goes, was from the land of Uz. He was upright and God-fearing, had ten children, seven thousand sheep, three thousand camels and a very large estate. The Bible tells us that Job was "wealthier than anyone in the East." But Job lost it all. Through an odd wager between God and Satan, Job became a helpless pawn in a divine scheme. Satan questioned God: if the blessed are truly loyal but lose everything, will they remain faithful? God replied in the affirmative and used Job to demonstrate the test. Loyal believers will retain their faith even at the cost of it all.

Without waiting to get through chapter 1, enemies plundered Job's animals, and a terrible wind collapsed on the house of his eldest son when all his siblings were feasting there, killing every last one. By the last verses of the chapter, Job has pulled out his hair and torn his clothes.

Bewildered, Job spent dozens of chapters perseverating on the issue of theodicy. He was doubted by friends who, instead of comforting him, reminded him that people who get punished must have done something wrong. Job questioned his own place in the universe and why he was ever born for such a fate. The sages of the Talmud believed that Job was a fictional character. They knew that the tragedy of Job's lot did exist in unfortunate numbers, and, living through the Roman persecutions and the destruction of their holy Temple, these scholars were on close terms with suffering. They could not believe, however, that such a wager would ever take place in a fair world. The story could never be real.

In the end, Job's quest for wisdom led him to a direct confrontation with the greatest human limitation: he could not access an understanding of death because he only had a slim glimmer of what the end looks like, a report created by Abandon and Death:

> But whence does wisdom come?
> Where is the source of understanding?
> It is hidden from the eyes of all living.
> Concealed from the fowl of heaven.
> Abandon and Death say
> "We have only a report of it."[1]

Job, like all of us, could never truly understand death with the intimacy of a "participant." He could only wait for a report, since even birds that soar in heaven have no access to this type of intelligence. Only Death can report on wisdom, since death inspires people to act more wisely.

Job was greatly diminished by his losses, but they eventually came to define and strengthen him. The very last chapter reports the reward for Job's well-oiled faith and his newly acquired wisdom: "The Lord gave Job twice what he had before" (42:10). Then the biblical text spells out the literal particulars if you can't do the math: fourteen thousand sheep, six thousand camels, et cetera. God replaced Job's ten children with ten more, in the exact gender set as before, on the assumption that children need not be doubled to offer compensatory joy. The very last words of the story? "So Job died old and contented" (42:17). Some may find this conclusion too happy even for a book on happy endings. Some may find it unrealistic. There are certain things that can never be replaced, like children. But perhaps the material wealth that was given in double the abundance was really a physical reflection of a metaphysical boon. Job had more because his close encounter with death enlarged his person, in every sense of the word.

We who read Job marvel at his resilience but would answer with a curt "no thanks" to the same offer. We'll forfeit the wisdom—thank you very much—to live without the tragedy. How, in the absence of death, should we acquire the wisdom that comes along with death's closest contact?

Many religions have contemplated the question and come up with symbols and rituals, stories and sayings to offer us the wisdom earned without the severe price: the easy-pass option, if you will. In both the Hindu and Buddhist traditions, a mandala (which means "circle" in Sanskrit) is a tool for meditation. It is usually a picture of a circle in a square enclosure, often made out of sand in intricate patterns that symbolize wholeness and harmony. Often a mandala is broken after days or weeks of adding to its intricacy, with all its sand scattered for its blessings to spread, to demonstrate the impermanence of life. The mandala helps people detach from this world to realize the fragility of life; all that we create over a lifetime can be smashed in only a moment. Take good care to never waste a moment. Everything is impermanent.

The Talmud, too, records a story of a celebration where people forgot how vulnerable life is and needed a dramatic reminder: "Mar, the son of Ravina, made a wedding for his son. He saw that the rabbis were getting too merry so he took a glass that was valued at four hundred zuz [a very large amount] and broke it in front of them, and they sobered up."[2] Mar was the life of the party, in a real sense, because he injected a moment of realism into the celebration.

Intricate sand paintings and expensive crystal goblets are used here as—to borrow a Latin expression—*memento mori*, physical reminders of death. The expression, which literally means "remember you will die," refers to a cluster of items and artwork designed as daily cues to prompt thoughts of mortality. We've all seen beautiful still-life paintings marred by a bizarre skull with darkened eye sockets on the table next to the fruit and flowers. That's a *memento mori*. Look at this, know you will die and do something meaningful as a result. Religion is designed to create a meaningful portal into the next world by enhancing the meaning of now. Mindfulness tells us that all we have is the very moment we are in. Nothing else is guaranteed.

A. J. Heschel, the rabbi and spiritualist, understood that death has a way of questioning every assumption we have about life. "In the presence of death there is only silence, and a sense of awe."[3] When we get over the shock and anger at death, we allow ourselves to be present in its mystery. Within faith traditions, silence and awe are complemented with a system of goodness to help us make each moment special, a system that enhances the transcendence of it all. Frame each day with rituals so that time is a blessing rather than a curse. Seek meaning as a worthwhile distraction. Do acts of kindness

Death gives every flat surface texture, every interchange the electricity of gravitas and every opportunity a sense of breathlessness. The *carpe diem* of graduation speeches means less when you reach out your arms to the world at twenty-one than when you grab the day at eighty-one, because at eighty-one there is a slow leak and that leak is the days left on your calendar. For this reason, we play with death, feigning lack of interest, thinking it a subject of little intrigue but wanting desperately to be let inside its secrets. Sherwin Nuland in *How We Die* captures this fascination well:

> To most people, death remains a hidden secret, as eroticized as it is feared. We are irresistibly attracted by the very anxieties we find most terrifying; we are drawn to them by a primitive excitement that arises from flirtation with danger. Moths and flames, mankind and death— there is little difference.[4]

The attraction/repulsion factor of death that Nuland captures is often at the heart of the human dialectic. We sway between living it up (the Talmudic partygoers) and toning it down (the broken sand painting that symbolizes human fragility). Religion tries to make the most of this dialectic by forcing us to act with goodness and compassion.

For two and a half years, two first-century giants of the Talmud argued about whether or not life was worth living. Shammai argued that it was better for human beings not to be created. Hillel argued that human beings were worth creating. After years of debate they compromised and agreed that life was not worth it, but that as long as we are alive, it is important to make the most of that life. Making the most of that life includes making the most of death.[5]

Enter the great Ecclesiastes/Epicurus debate.

King Solomon, the author of Ecclesiastes according to traditional views, began a search for life's purpose and created a living laboratory to test out every thesis. "I put my mind to studying, exploring, and seeking wisdom and the reason of things, and to studying wickedness, stupidity, madness and folly" (7:25). *Kohelet*, the Hebrew name of the book, is from the root word for "gathering." Some believe that the term refers to a preacher or a teacher, but it seems more likely that *kohelet* refers less to the one who gathers the aphorisms than the collected gathering of sayings itself that resulted from his various experiments. The wealthiest of Israelite kings, Solomon spared no expense in his search. He purchased excessive property and surrounded himself with luxury, but in this he found no lasting comfort or pleasure: "I multiplied my possessions. I built myself houses and planted vineyards. I laid out gardens and groves, in which I planted every kind of fruit tree. . . . I got enjoyment out of all my wealth. And that was all I got out of my wealth" (2:4–10). He immersed himself in love and lust but to no enduring end: "Now I find woman more bitter than death;

she is all traps, her hands are fetters and her heart is snares" (7:26). He tested it all but to no avail.

Our pious narrator partied until he discovered that that was futile too: "I said to myself, 'Come I will treat you to merriment. Taste mirth!' That, too, I found was futile. Of revelry I said, 'It's mad.' Of merriment, 'What good is that?'" (2:1–2). He began to hate his life. He went back to eating and drinking and advised his readers to do that with all of their means as long as they know that it all comes from God. He argued that there is nothing new under the sun and that all is vanity: "All I tested with wisdom, O thought I could fathom it, but it eludes me. The secret of what happens is elusive and deep, deep down; who can discover it?" (7:23–24). Solomon had arrived at Job's conclusion but without the pain.

Ecclesiastes is pockmarked with hypocrisies and contradictions. At times, the narrator is upbeat and hopeful. His wallowing in wealth and physical pleasures taught him to see these distractions for what they were: temporary pleasure. He questioned the transitory nature of life and believed that only wisdom had endurance. He concluded that there is a time for everything: "A time for being born and a time for dying, a time for planting and a time for uprooting the planted" (3:1–2). The uncertainty of death inspired Solomon to greater adherence to law and a life of wisdom-seeking, and the second to last verse of the book is repeated in synagogue during liturgical readings: "The sum of the matter, when all is said and done: Revere God and observe his commandments for this is the totality of mankind" (12:13). Some scholars believe that Solomon or the unnamed narrator never ended this way. It was a flourish by others, tacking a note of purpose to an otherwise existentially cynical book whose inclusion in the biblical canon was debated vigorously. It was a happy ending to distract the reader from the otherwise wearying conclusion that life has little purpose.

I believe this reading is a mistake and fails to entertain the contradictory aspects of the book, which mirror the contradictory aspects of life. We rise. We fall. We feel winded. We feel bloated with glee. We arrive at conclusions about the nature of life and our purpose from an amalgamation of experiences that do not fit neatly together. "But man sets out for his eternal abode, with mourners all around in the street. . . . And the dust returns to the ground as it was, and the lifebreath returns to God Who bestowed it" (12:5–7). We are only stewards of this life, and our custodial responsibilities to wisdom, relationships and piety are many. We are confused. I am confused.

On the journey to wisdom, Solomon concluded that there *is* a destination. Swinging between hedonism and his own desire for wisdom and goodness, he arrived at a middle ground: enjoying life's material pleasures and wisdom while knowing that it is all from God.

> Go eat your bread in gladness, and drink your wine in joy; for your action was long ago approved by God. . . . Enjoy happiness with the woman you love all the fleeting days of your life that have been granted to you under the sun—all your fleeting days. For that alone is what you can get out of life and out of the means you acquire under the sun. Whatever is in your power to do, do with all your might. For there is not action, no reason, no learning, no wisdom in Sheol, where you are going (9:7–10).

Even when Solomon did not specifically mention death, the allusions to it are abundant. The fleeting nature of time and experience is repeated chapter after chapter. Realizing that the wise man and the fool both meet the same end, Solomon understood that dying is the only experience that can measure out the true meaning of a life. Take risks since you do not know your end: "Sow your seed in the morning, and don't hold back your hand in the evening since you don't know which is going to succeed" (11:6). Make the most of this life because at its end there is no action, no reason, no learning, no wisdom. All of that can only be garnered right here and right now.

Solomon mentioned death explicitly as a method of learning to live, a fraught but genuine way to uncover life's priorities:

> It is better to go to the house of mourning, than to go to the house of feasting: for that is the end of all humanity; and the living will lay it to his heart. Sorrow is better than laughter: for by the sadness of the countenance the heart is made better. The heart of the wise is in the house of mourning; but the heart of fools is in the house of mirth. (Eccl. 7:2–4)

Some may not realize that Edith Wharton took a title for one of her books straight from Ecclesiastes. But her house of mirth was not Solomon's house of mourning. Quite the opposite. Solomon wanted us to learn death's lessons from a house of mourning rather than taking up Wharton's call to the life of trivial pursuits. Sober yourself up in a house of mourning, and you will overlay your heart with the truth: death is the end of all humanity. Sorrow humbles us. Mirth fools us. The wise leave their hearts in the house of mourning because that is where the heart learns to enlarge itself.

When I think of these verses, I connect them to my friend Josh's mother. In a seminar I taught, Josh shared a source of inspiration for his leadership: his mother. When Josh was twelve and his mother was about forty, doctors detected cancer and presented her with two options: aggressive chemotherapy that might or might not reduce the growth or an acceptance of cancer's terrible trajectory. She was determined to take on the cancer and opted for chemotherapy. At one point in her treatment, her physician told her that the chemotherapy was not working, and her death was imminent. She pulled Josh aside and told him that from that point forward, she intended to live each day as if it were a bonus. She would love harder, give more, do more. Today she is seventy-eight. By my count, she has had 13,870 bonus days, and by Josh's account, she's treated each one as a surprise.

Not everyone agrees about living each day as a present and making meaning every day because we will eventually die and are always advancing toward death. Where religion emphasizes the mystery of death, a good afterlife and days packed with goodness, existentialist philosophers take an entirely different tack. Not everyone takes the threat of death seriously or believes that death inspires us to enhanced living. Maybe it's best not to take death too seriously. Johnny Carson once joked that "for three days after death, hair and fingernails continue to grow, but phone calls taper off."

The existential philosopher Jean-Paul Sartre famously wrote about the vanity that Solomon captured but without the same conclusions:

> Death is never that which gives life its meaning; it is, on the contrary, that which on principle removes all meaning from life. If we must die, then our life has no meaning because its problems receive no solution and because the very meaning of the problems remains undetermined.[6]

How is that for meaninglessness? Sartre's resignation is not quite as tart as the dismissal of death offered by another Frenchman, Voltaire, who on his deathbed reputedly said in response to a priest who asked that he renounce Satan, "Now, now, my good man. This is no time for making enemies."

Voltaire's sarcasm captures a much earlier debate. The ancient Greek philosopher and hedonist Epicurus argues in his *Letter to Menoeceus* that death is "nothing to us." It does not enhance meaning; if anything, knowledge of death enhances the possibility of pleasure. "And therefore a right understanding that death is nothing to us makes the mortality of life enjoyable, not because it adds to it an infinite span of time, but because it takes away the craving for immortality."[7] Once we know that we will not live forever, we can recommit ourselves to a life of pleasure, argues the hedonist, because we know that nothing we do will have lasting impact. Here Epicurus is speaking strictly about the death of the body, since immortality can be achieved through memories, offspring, writings, works of art and other noncorporeal creations that outlive us. But he thought that if we let go of any expectation of immortality, we'd probably spend our time in this world in greater states of delight.

Epicurus did not believe that death is evil, since dead people cannot experience death and can, therefore, have no judgment about its moral qualities. Since death is not evil, and the dead cannot fear death, then *no one* should fear death:

> But the wise man does not fear the cessation of life, for neither does life offend him nor does the absence of life seem to be any evil. And just as with food he does not seek simply the larger share and nothing else, but rather the most pleasant, so he seeks to enjoy not the longest period of time, but the most pleasant.[8]

A short, delicious life would seem to the hedonist to be much preferred to a long life punctuated with suffering. Death is not an evil; it just is.

Some philosophers believe that death is not even an event in our lives because we are not alive to experience it as such. We have premonitions of death, fantasies about death and even near encounters with death. One thinker observes that "the state of death is comparable to a rendezvous that the human being keeps on missing."[9] We know that death will approach us at some date unknown to us, but the fact that we don't know the time of death offers an ever-present irritation. If we only had that information, we could be more planful. Maybe it's an event we *want* to keep missing so we avoid thinking about it. It's like those e-vites that we keep not opening. They sneak into our in-box at inconvenient times and force us to ask some unpleasant, confrontational questions of our limited calendars.

The Epicurus approach certainly challenges religious attitudes and behaviors around death. We find undertones of Epicurus in the oddest of places, like the sides of a red double-decker bus in London. In 2008–2009, the British Humanist Association, the comic writer Ariane Sherine and the evolutionary biologist Richard Dawkins created the "Atheist Bus Campaign," which involved plastering messages about atheism across buses and other forms of public transportation. Taking a cue from Epicurus, one poster, which appeared on thirty buses in London, read: "There's probably no God. Now stop worrying and enjoy your life." A number of Christian groups reacted strongly to these advertisements and launched opposing campaigns with their own slogans:

- "There definitely is a God; so join the Christian Party and enjoy your life."
- "The fool hath said in his heart, There is no God."[10]
- "There IS a God, BELIEVE. Don't worry and enjoy your life."

Faith is not the only issue under question in the bus mantra war. The slogans also hint at what drives happiness. Is it hedonism? It just doesn't matter, we're all going to die anyway. Or is it meaning? Because it *does* matter, *and* we're all going to die anyway.

The only problem is that death is a certainty, but the time of death remains uncertain, mortality clock notwithstanding. Epicurus uses this uncertainty to fuel a life of debauchery and excitement with each passing day. Uncertainty prompts pleasure. If you don't know how long you've got, party until you drop. Epicurus would have had an amazing fraternity house in college.

I was unsure how to resolve the Ecclesiastes/Epicurus debate. One day I was talking about the great debate with a friend, who told me that I must meet an acquaintance of his named Gaurov. Gaurov, he was sure, could help me in my quest. Gaurov was the chief medical officer for a health care system and a pediatrician by training. A Hindu whose name means "pride" or "respect" in Sanskrit, Gaurov turned forty this past year. But although his personal and professional life was flowering and stable, he began to experience some odd neurological symptoms that exposed him to a brief, almost fatal scare:

> As a physician myself I blew it off but then things got progressively worse. A few months later, I had an extensive work-up, maybe seven or eight physicians were trying to figure this out, and I had hundreds of tests. I had neurological instability and difficulty walking. My heart raced when I walked. I had feelings of heat and would wake up drenched in sweat. My ankles were swelling, and I would flush. It was gradually getting worse and then one week I couldn't stand up, and I knew something was really wrong.

Gaurov describes himself as a rational person, driven by scientific research. His faith background also informs his life spiritually, but in this instance, the fear of death was hitting Gaurov as a medical rather than a religious event, driving one side of his brain rather than the other. He speaks of the time of his illness and his symptoms with dispassion and a slight remove, almost as if all of his troubles happened to someone else. "I don't know if I was dying. I thought I was for a while."

He acknowledges that the delivery of his near-death narrative might sound mechanical but explains that he and his wife, who is also a physician, searched the internet and spoke with people to get to the bottom of the condition. They treated Gaurov's symptoms as intellectual problems to be solved. "I looked things up and thought it was likely this or that, but also, in the back of my mind, I was thinking that it could be really bad—possibly MS or cancer."

Gaurov was about to go on a family vacation to Greece with his wife, his five-year-old daughter and his parents. The day before he left, an oncologist friend of his sat him down in his office and said that, based on his symptoms, he likely had metastasized cancer and in all likelihood had about eighteen months to live. Gaurov recalls that the doctor was pretty confident in the diagnosis, and although Gaurov understood that cancer was a likely suspect, he didn't realize the full extent of his condition until he left the office and began researching the diagnosis.

> Even at that point, in the back of my mind I thought it's not the worst thing in the world. But when I started doing my research I saw just how bad this was going to be. I cursed and then talked to my wife, but both of us had more of a "this isn't good" reaction because what the doctor suspected I had was not confirmed either. But that's when my thinking started changing. I realized this really could be my last vacation. The survival rate was very poor.

Gaurov told friends and family what was going on. As a physician he deals with life and death all of the time, but he realized then that it was always in the context of someone else's health. He was not afraid for himself. His only fears were related to how others would handle the news. He worried about his parents. He worried that his five-year-old daughter would be too young to have a lot of memories of him. He wanted her to get to know him, and he wanted to know her. But that looked increasingly impossible.

When Gaurov told people at work, his secretary started bawling. No one understood why he was still going on vacation, but he felt that if he was going to die, he might as well take a great vacation with his family. What difference did it make now if he stayed or went? He made a list of things he had to do. Making the list helped him realize that he had traveled a lot and really had done a lot of what he wanted to do in this world. "My list wasn't long," Gaurov said with a laugh, "I'd been living a good life." If he died the next day, he would be a happy, blessed man. "When I started thinking in terms of a year or two years, I began to think I'd do anything to get a decade. Ten years seemed like forever. But if you ask me now, ten years seems like nothing." His perceptions of time changed when he thought he was living and when he thought he was dying.

The trip was good for him. The plane ride was also a gift. The flight was fourteen hours, and everyone was asleep. Gaurov wasn't disturbed by e-mails and cellphone calls and could just think about the momentousness of this time in his life. He says sheepishly that there was one thing that he really wanted, and he decided on that trip that he was going to get it. "It sounds so cliché, but I always wanted a sports car, and in Greece I began to look up sports cars on the internet. We came back on a Saturday night, and by Sunday I was at a car dealership." This wasn't a pure impulse buy for Gaurov. He had been thinking about it as his fortieth birthday rolled around. He figured he'd probably own one within the next five years, but his diagnosis collapsed the wait, and he decided to go for it. "That's another thing this taught me: if you want to do something, just do it."

So far, Gaurov's reaction to his imminent death was taking on an Epicurean overtone. Vacation. Sports car. A "what does it matter?" attitude. Epicurus had just found himself another disciple. In fact, because he was vacationing in Greece, I even thought to myself that he could have visited Samos, the Aegean island where Epicurus was born. Yet the brief separation from Gaurov's work and his everyday life while in Greece only augmented the tension of what lay in store for him upon his return.

What would his prognosis now mean in terms of work, his family, his short future? Decisions mounted. How long would he be able to keep up his practice? What would this mean for his wife, who herself had a busy physician's career? What should he say and do in light of the fact that his life was soon to be over, and his young daughter might never even remember him?

Gaurov had a nuclear scan scheduled for right after his trip. He got back Saturday night. Being a doctor, he had a crop of health care professionals at his disposal, something that just doesn't materialize for the average patient. By Wednesday he knew that he did not have cancer. He immediately texted his wife the good news. The oncologist who had given him the original diagnosis practically shrugged off the mistake. Gaurov didn't blame him for the emotional havoc the diagnosis wreaked on the family. Medicine is an art and a science. People make mistakes. They're just trying to do their jobs as well as they can. "Well, if this isn't it, let's figure out what you do have," the doctor said, and Gaurov followed his lead. Being a physician himself helped him put the mistake into perspective. There are margins of error built into every discipline, and Gaurov's reprieve was the best outcome he could have wanted. It seemed unlikely for him to get angry at being told that he was now going to live, having gone to the most profound place of despair with his family only days before.

•  •  •

He kept the sports car.

Despite the changes and chaos of those months, Gaurov said the real hit came a few weeks later. In the beginning of May he was told the good news that his illness was not life-threatening. A month later, his otherwise healthy brother-in-law died in a motorcycle accident. Three days before the accident, Gaurov and his brother-in-law went on a road trip. They spent a lot of time talking about Gaurov's diagnosis and how it affected him and the family. His brother-in-law wanted to know what he was thinking and feeling.

> And now I look back on that time, and here I was talking all about myself and death and then three days later, my totally healthy brother-in-law is dead, leaving behind a wife and three teenagers. Their oldest son has metastasized cancer, so when I called people about my brother-in-law, everyone thought I meant my nephew. That shook me up. It was so random. Life is very fragile, and it's amazing how someone can be here and then be gone. And life goes on.

Those who were supposed to die lived, and those who were supposed to live died. It all shook Gaurov up. It's as if a divine sort of havoc set in, and he was walking through it, not knowing if there was an exit sign anywhere nearby.

Gaurov's faith only complicated matters. He has a strong belief that we shouldn't make deals with God when things go wrong, promising that we'll increase our good deeds or our charity just because we want to purchase God's good graces when things are rough. But he had a hard time grappling with why so many things started to fall apart in his life in such a short time span. It's not that he found himself doubting God, but he realized that he had more unanswered questions than before and was pulling away from religion. He practiced less. It stopped being a source of comfort for him. Perhaps his faith had been too simplistic to hold the new uncertainty that was now his lot.

But unlike Epicurus, Gaurov interpreted the presence of death in his life as a transformative experience, one he is still trying to understand. He doesn't believe he is a changed person totally, as we might expect of someone who undergoes this kind of shake-up. Maybe the quick time frame in which he was told he was going to die and then told he was going to live did not offer him the time to settle into either prospect in depth. But his was not a shallow encounter either. Philosophically, he believes that we are who we are no matter the circumstances:

> For me, one of the things that really impacted me is to make the most of what I have. I'm very focused on work. Work has always been important to me, but now I am much more intentional. I keep asking myself and my boss, Does what I'm doing really matter? Is it creating something of value? Am I doing something worthwhile? I think I'm also doing more things. Here's a trivial example. Last week I rented a sailboat and went sailing with friends and family. It's not a big deal, but I probably wouldn't have done it a few months ago, before all this happened.

Gaurov's commitment to family was solid and stable and not subject to the vagaries of experience. What changed the most for Gaurov by channeling in and out of dying was his attitude about work and play. On the one hand, he was able to let go of the intensity of work and its demands. The freedom of the wind in the sails of a boat filled with friends was a luxury he would probably have denied himself before. Now he gave himself these small, pleasurable interruptions, like Solomon telling us to enjoy a glass of wine. On the other hand, Gaurov's sense of purposefulness about what he did shifted from familial and personal expectations of professional success to seeing his role as a healer and as someone who was able to enhance life and bring life to others through medicine. Not everyone goes into medicine to heal others. Many go into the field for medicine's perceived prestige or out of family or personal pressure or as a statement of intelligence or for the financial stability. Speaking to Gaurov, it was as if he was only now actualizing what medicine could really become ideologically when his own life faced a sudden end and then he welcomed life again. It was like getting another chance to try something on for its fit when the fit, this time, would be much more personally descriptive and prescriptive. Medicine, for Gaurov, went from a job to a calling.

But when I put his experience to him in the context of Epicurus versus Ecclesiastes, Gaurov rejected the dichotomy.

> I want to do more good work *and* I want to have more fun. . . . Have no fear. Make sure that what you're doing is valuable. I definitely haven't gone down the path of debauchery, but I'm looking to enjoy life more, and for me that isn't just related to driving a faster car. It's also enjoyment of work and personal life. We still don't know what it is that I have—probably some unexplainable neurological illness—so I have daily reminders of my disease that help me keep a positive attitude.

Gaurov wasn't transforming his life as a result of his encounter with death. He was deepening it. Everything he was doing he continued to do, but at a more intense pace and level. While the depth of his life has increased, it has also slowed down. A year ago Gaurov ran a marathon. Now, he says, he could never do that. His body is teaching him to accept a new self, one that has not yet crossed to safety, to borrow from Wallace Stegner, when it comes to neurological health. His health scare left residual health-related problems, but these have made Gaurov a more compassionate physician:

> I learned something about the health care system being a patient. I felt when I was sick that no one was in charge of my health. I realized that we have to make a more patient-centric system. . . . We focus on doctors, but our job should be to focus on helping patients get through things. I think our system is very broken, but now I'm more focused on doing something about it than talking about it.

Gaurov had the means and the network to cope with his diagnosis, surrounded as he was by family members and friends who are doctors. Needing the care of the system, he began to realize its holes once on the other side. He has crossed back but not totally, which has enabled him to see the anguish of patients who lack advocates and find themselves suddenly thrown into the sterile world of medical terminology without the tenderness and nurturing that patients need when vulnerable. If he can change a little piece of the system, then his own scare will have offered important dividends.

Gaurov is still in the thick of processing the past months. Some of the ideas he has now about changing the health care system may become weaker over time, as the pall of death moves farther away and his close visit with cancer recedes into the background. But for now, he carries the lessons of both Epicurus and Ecclesiastes with him: "One constant theme I had playing in my head is that life is very valuable. You only appreciate it when it's gone, not when you have it. When it starts slipping away, you realize it. Life is so valuable. My goal is to not forget that. I've gone to the edge and stepped back a little, but I can still see it. That's my goal—to not forget that."

●　　●　　●

After spending time with Gaurov, I realized that I had not actually put the question to myself: Ecclesiastes or Epicurus? As a teacher of the Bible, I find Ecclesiastes is a friend. It is one of my favorite books, packed as it is with ancient wisdom and even more ancient life contradictions. It humanizes the Bible and somehow always catches me in the tailspin of my own faith struggles with goodness and mortality. But I was also a philosophy major in college, and while Epicurus and I did not party together (I don't think I even got invited to a party in college), I knew where he stood, and I appreciated his stance. I appreciate it more with age, after leaving funerals or hearing bad news and trying to get a large gulp of air in my system and leave some heaviness behind. Do girls just want to have fun? Sometimes we need to. I am aware that there are sad movies that are great movies that I will probably never see because, on the few occasions when I go to movies, I want an escape. As I make more casseroles for more friends with cancer, I've taken a shallower view of happiness. It looks more like a steaming cup of tea at four in the afternoon and the cool feel of the sheets when I first get into bed at night.

For me, a persistent chaser of meaning and inspiration, I used to find the encounter with death more of a life prompter when I experienced less of it personally. I would read of a terrible catastrophe and work harder, teach more hours, hug the kids more and force the most out of each day. I worked with a kind of spiritual propulsion. Time was a constant foe.

As I age and have lost friends and family members, I am less interested in productivity and more interested in relationships. Everything for me now is not about a fast grab to make something new; it's a slow dance where I hope to hold on to love and trust and enjoy it as long as possible. It's Ecclesiastes turned Epicurus and back again.

And I realized in posing the question to myself—Ecclesiastes or Epicurus—that it is not about one or the other but about the shuffle we engage in as we move cautiously between them.

I heard about a family that did just that. They shuffled between Ecclesiastes and Epicurus, and they learned to use one death to make the next death better.

Mike is the son of Greta and Fred, two hardworking parents who, before they retired, managed a store. Mike dropped out of college in his third year, not because he wasn't smart but because the treadmill of classes semester after semester wasn't working, and he didn't want to be in school anymore. He wasn't sure what he wanted out of life. From the moment he left college, Mike and Fred began an embattled relationship. Mike was their only son, and Fred held him up to a high standard. He was always telling people who Mike could have been: he could have been this. He could have been that, and, like a pesky school report card, he summed up Mike's condition: he was not achieving his potential. When Fred became ill, Mike did his best to be there for his dad, but there was a huge and impenetrable chasm between them. It was hard for Mike to give back to a man who constantly diminished him, especially a parent.

Greta was always running interference between husband and son. She did not want her husband to feel disrespected, and she certainly didn't want to alienate her son. She saw the price of disappointment in their relationship. Instead, Greta specialized in shuttle diplomacy.

Fred's disease spread. His speech became slurred, and he was increasingly hard to understand. He was frustrated because the words formed in his head, but he lacked the ability to articulate them. Greta was the only person who could understand him. Soon he was going to lose the capacity to speak altogether while retaining his mental faculties. He knew, Greta knew and Mike knew that the end was nearing, but reconciliation was not. Greta broke down one evening and shared the difficulty between the two with a rabbi who came to visit the couple often. She couldn't bear the tension anymore, or the fact that if the problem went unresolved, they would soon lose the chance to resolve it.

The rabbi was a seasoned professional when it came to pastoral care, as if he had an honorary doctorate in compassion. Rabbi Miller complained to me that too many clergy today have forgotten the simple art of kindness in favor of scholarship. When he vacationed he would make sure to send postcards to every single widow in his congregation. His was an aging congregation, and this small gesture meant so much that his list of recipients kept growing. It became so onerous that he soon had to write and stamp them before he went away. Rabbi Miller helped me understand why the help of a third party, especially someone with spiritual credentials, can be critical in prompting deathbed reconciliation when the "warring" parties simply lack the tools to help themselves.

The rabbi said that he sensed tension in the father/son dynamic but did not know the extent until Greta opened up. They both knew how much Mike needed the reconciliation, but they also knew that it had to come from Fred. Mike had decided to lead his own life. He was not going to say to his father, "I'm sorry I failed you. I'm sorry I picked my own path." Mike's self-esteem was severely compromised; he was only in his early thirties but felt stunted. "Rabbi, is there anything you can do?" Greta pleaded. Rabbi Miller offered to talk to Fred.

The rabbi went into Fred's room alone and pulled up a chair next to his bed. "Fred, I know you love Mike. You have to make it right now because if you don't, you're going to reach a point soon where you will not be able to, and you know you won't be able to. The ideas will be trapped in your brain, and you will not be able to express them. You will not have words. And that will be the worst hell of all. Beyond that, you don't want to leave this earth with unfinished business, and the only unfinished business you have on this planet right now is between you and Mike. It's fairly irrelevant if you were right or if Mike was right. What we need now, Fred, is *shalom*, peace." Rabbi Miller explained to Fred that the root of *shalom* in Hebrew is *shalem*, "to be whole," "to be complete." The rabbi was straightforward and did not mince his words: "Fred, we have to make this right. I need your permission. I want to tell Mike that you'd like to have a moment with him."

The rabbi had trouble understanding Fred by this point, and he saw in front of him a man tangled in language who could only haltingly get a few words out. In a very difficult way, Fred was trying to let out all kinds of feelings when the rabbi tasked him with confronting Mike. Rabbi Miller confessed that he didn't really understand Fred at this point but felt that maybe he didn't need to. He realized that he just needed to listen to him. "I guessed that he was granting me permission, but I really didn't know. I asked him again, "Can I just ask Mike to come in? Can you get two words out: 'I'm sorry'? And then three words: 'I love you'? Just five words. Can you do it?"

Rabbi Miller began to cry as he told me the story. He paused, blew his nose and then returned to that room where a family drama was about to unfold.

Fred started to cry. Tears are stronger than words. Fred nodded his affirmation. Yes. He did want time alone with Mike. The rabbi left the room and casually said, "Mike, your dad wants to see you." Mike was confused. He looked at the rabbi incredulously. He asked his mom to come in, perhaps feeling anxious about the encounter, but the rabbi made fast eye contact with Greta, and she understood. Mike went in alone. Five minutes passed. Ten minutes passed. Greta looked at the rabbi and said, "They haven't spent this much time alone together since

Mike was a kid." Forty-five minutes later, Mike left Fred's bedside. With tears in his eyes, he looked at his mother and said, "Dad loves me."


Rabbi Miller paused again, "I watched Greta die in the same bed Fred died in." The words hung in the air before the rabbi explained.

Greta forgave people easily. Because she worked in retail sales and dealt with tough customers, she would say, "You never know what the whole story is." She met all kinds of people; they needed advice or help or were simply looking for company. She also lived with a husband who held grudges and nursed wounds, and she had watched him die. Greta forgave people throughout her life. She often said, "No one is perfect," and she let herself live comfortably around imperfection, perhaps because her own life was never easy. Or maybe she had watched what Fred's intolerance had done to him and his relationship with Mike, and she made a conscious point of being accepting and tolerant.

After Fred died, Greta wanted to get on with her life. Through the period of caregiving, she had taken an Ecclesiastes approach to death. She wanted ends to be tied up and the relationships to heal. She wanted to do what was right in the face of Fred's death. And just as Ecclesiastes preached, "There is a time to be born and a time to die," Greta went through death and then wanted to live a little. She was in her eighties and wanted to do things she hadn't done for years; as Fred's caregiver, she had hardly allowed herself any indulgence. Now she wanted to go to the movies, go to a show, go to Atlantic City and gamble. Since Fred couldn't enjoy these activities with her, she had not done them in years. Her life revolved around him. Within a few months of Fred's death, she too needed permission: permission to live, to make new friends and to spend time with old friends. Epicurus was making a comeback. After a long hiatus, Greta was finally able to enjoy herself.

One day a little over a year after Fred died, Greta wasn't feeling well. After a series of tests, the results came back positive: she had pancreatic cancer. Greta decided that she would be in charge of her own life as much as possible. She wanted to know the treatment options and wanted to be treated only if it would prolong a quality life, but she did not want what had happened to Fred. She went through a round of chemo. It was difficult, but she remained upbeat and determined. The rabbi and Greta had a thumbs-up sign between them to signal that Greta was okay. She even used it with him when he visited her in intensive care. After the first round of chemo, she decided to do as many things as she could and withhold medical treatment. She was pushing Epicurus to the limit. She used to worry if she'd have enough money to live on and enough to pass on to the kids. Greta was a frugal woman, but at the end of her life, she taught herself to splurge. She went out to dinner by herself once a week. She bought what she wanted without holding back as she once would have. She was determined to enjoy every day that she had left.

After a few months, weak and somewhat defeated, she went to the hospital. The doctors were split in their opinions on Greta's treatment plan. One doctor wanted to pursue aggressive treatment, and another felt that Greta shouldn't be in pain in her last months. She had already lost her hair after the chemo, but it started to come back. Greta needed regular blood transfusions every one to two weeks. After the transfusion, she'd feel a lot better, but it was clear that her condition was worsening. The rabbi continued to visit her regularly, and once, when he was slated to lecture in Canada, he saw Greta and told her he would be away for eleven days. "She wanted to know exactly when I was leaving and exactly when I was getting back. She asked me several times when I was getting back, even though she knew I was going to be away for eleven days." Perhaps Greta understood how near she was to her life's end, because eight days into Rabbi Miller's trip, Greta's daughter called: "Rabbi, Mom took a turn for the worse yesterday. When exactly are you going to be back?"

Three days. The rabbi heard real concern in Greta's daughter's voice and decided to call Greta. Greta's voice was weak. She asked the rabbi once again when he was coming back, and to the answer "Three days," she responded by saying that she had to look at her calendar. "It's a little more than forty-eight hours, so after you rest up, would it be okay for us to see each other?" The rabbi was planning to visit but made a last-minute decision to go to Greta's home straight from the airport.

> I had a strong sense that Greta was not going to die until I got back, so I didn't want to curtail the trip. She said she wanted me to be there with her kids and give her eulogy. I can't explain it, but I had a sense that she was going to live, and if I shortened the trip she would die earlier. I got there. The whole family was there. Her three kids came from all around the country. The house had the feeling of a death vigil. The kids were pacing, taking turns going in and out of Greta's bedroom. I walked in, and Greta was dozing. There was a rolling tray table so that she could eat. A helper from hospice was there. I said to her daughter, "Your mom looks peaceful. Maybe I'll come back later."

Rabbi Miller thought he would go home, see his wife, wash up and go back, but Greta's daughter, Rachel, was insistent. Greta had given her unambiguous directions: "If and when the rabbi comes, wake me up." Rachel gently whispered to her mother that the rabbi was in the living room. Greta wanted to see him. She was very fragile, but she managed to lift up her thumb, their special sign, when he came into the room.

"Would you please do me a favor, Rabbi?"

"Greta, whatever you want."

"Please go into the dining room with Mike. In the bottom of the breakfront, behind some tablecloths, I want you to get something and bring it to me. It's hidden. There is a bottle of champagne. Would you please bring that bottle here and would you ask Mike to bring us six champagne glasses?"

The rabbi left and gave Mike his instructions. Mike replied, "There is no champagne in this house, Rabbi. My mother doesn't drink."

"I don't know what to tell you. Your mother said there is a bottle of champagne in the breakfront." Sure enough, it was there. It was an old bottle of champagne that had been back there for a long time. The children were confused. The rabbi brought in the champagne. Mike brought in the glasses. Greta asked to be propped up. She had a hard time swallowing, and at this stage she could only drink small sips of liquid through a straw. Greta smiled. "Rabbi, would you please open up the bottle of champagne?"

Now the rabbi was confused. There were five people in the room: Greta, three children and himself, yet Greta wanted six glasses. "Yes, Greta, but can you please tell me why we're opening this bottle of champagne and why you need six glasses?" As weak as she was, Greta was loud and coherent enough so that all the children could hear. "Fred and I bought that champagne on our twenty-fifth wedding anniversary. We decided we were going to open it on our fiftieth wedding anniversary. But Fred didn't make it. I want you to pour six glasses — one for Fred — and put a straw in one glass for me." Everyone in the room was speechless. The rabbi asked Greta if she wanted to make a blessing on the wine, but she asked the rabbi to do it. He said the blessing, as Greta looked up and said, "Before you drink, say *L'chaim*: 'To life!'" Greta had suffered through Fred's miserable death and decided, instead, to take the champagne route. She used her husband's death to teach her how to live and then to show her how *not* to die. She saw in him resignation but not inspiration, and she was determined to do death differently.

Then Greta made her own blessing, the *Shehekhiyanu*, a blessing traditionally recited at milestone events and occasions of happiness and significance: "Blessed are you, O Lord, King of the Universe, who has sustained us, nurtured us and allowed us to live to this day."

Greta continued with a blessing of her own making: "Thank you, God, for bringing me to this day. I lived to see my children grow up. I lived to see good grandchildren. I was married to a good man, and I have everything to be thankful and grateful for." Greta then gave the traditional children's blessing recited on the Sabbath to her son and daughters. She sighed and said, "I am really tired. I would just like to rest now for a little while." And with a look of angelic peace, Greta put her head down on the pillow.

Rabbi Miller was flummoxed. "I've accompanied people in their last moments of life for so many years, dozens and dozens of times. In my whole career, of all the deaths I've witnessed, I've never heard someone say a blessing over their own death."

Greta's breathing was stable, not labored or shallow as it so often is when a person is on the brink of death. Rachel sat by her bed and recited psalms. When Rabbi Miller saw Greta lying peacefully, he told the children that he would be back shortly. After all, he had not seen his own wife and children yet. An hour later, he got a call. Greta, filled with gratitude, having enjoyed champagne sipped through a straw and the blessings of a full life, had passed on from this world.

# Epilogue

A close friend called to tell me that her grandmother had died two months shy of her ninety-seventh birthday. At her funeral, my friend rang with praise: "Grandma, you were always right; you were always first and were always the best at everything. And even if you weren't, you believed you were." And that described her last moments in a hospital bed. Her two sons flanked the bed and each held one hand. In the room were the cast of characters who peopled her life: her grandchildren, daughters-in-law, great-grandchildren. They all said goodbye. They prayed with her and sang "A Woman of Valor" together, the verses of which are nestled in the last chapter of the biblical book of Proverbs. And then her son said that it was time, and she closed her eyes and breathed her last. *Let that be me,* I whispered to God when I hung up the phone.

*Ah, I thought, a happier ending.* Happy endings are usually reserved for fairy tales; they are rarely the stuff of our lives. But sometimes we get lucky. As I age and redefine and renegotiate the terms, semi-happiness seems to be a good enough deal. I'll take it. I've slowly adjusted to life's nuances and, on a good day, may even feel blessed precisely because not everything is happy. I have come to understand that in a life punctured with sadness, there can be satisfaction, growth and resilience. There is love.

## *Be prepared.*

I have written my ethical will. I'm not going to lie to you: it was arduous. I was teary at times, but if I thought it was important to do before I wrote it, I think it's exponentially more important to have now that it's done. It made me strip myself bare and think about what I have not compromised on in this lifetime. It was an exercise in values like no other. Happy reading, kids.

And I did buy a burial plot for two. It was retail. I thought that alone was going to kill me. They always have secondhand plots for sale in newspapers, but why is someone selling their plot anyway? It's not used. That's weird.

It had to be done. I'd rather choose the place than have it chosen for me last minute under the haze of loss and confusion. We did have to pay in advance—which always hurts—but I hope that it represents an overall savings if the price of real estate goes up (which they are predicting). I've made my burial wishes explicit in the ethical will. You can thank me for that too, kids. One less thing to fight about.

I haven't said all my "sorrys" yet. One lifetime may not be enough to accomplish that. From so many people I spoke to I learned the cost secondhand of not being forgiving, and I won't soon forget it.

I've learned a lot more than that. We can rage against death and fight illnesses until they squeeze the life out of us. We can act as fugitives from death's grip. We can give away our material possessions before we go and share advice with the living. We can take care of the messy, unfinished business of words not said. We can apologize and overcome our fears. We can even write a book about death. None of it will stay the angel of death's visit. It will just mean that in a universe where so little is in our control, we are ready for a happier ending.

*I am ready.*

*Appendix*

# Writing an Ethical Will

Why do people write ethical wills? We write them to make our deepest wishes and values known. We write them to be remembered. We write them because we realize that our wisdom and life experience are our most important legacy and sometimes our only legacy. We write ethical wills to bless others and become more aware of our own blessings. This sense of abundance envelops us with a sense of fullness and gratitude. It enables us to celebrate life, even when the end of life may be painful and grim. It offers a grand retrospective on what our lives have been all about, what has shaped us and what we have shaped over the course of a lifetime. The writing of an ethical will can help us age with a greater sense of dignity as we sift out priorities and what has been essential to living well, and what has not. It helps us confront mistakes and regrets. It offers us self-worth and accomplishment, and it can help provide completion to the writer and direction to the reader.

Basically, ethical wills answer three central questions:

- Do those I care about know what is most important to me and what I've learned through experience?
- Have I said everything that I need to say to my family and friends?
- Do those nearest and dearest to me know my burial wishes?

If this kind of clarity is helpful to the dying, why don't more people write ethical wills? For one thing, it forces us to contemplate our end, and no one wants to write something that assumes one's nonexistence. An ethical will is a summative document; it asks us to think of our most important values, and we might not feel ready to make those kinds of grandiose statements.

Practically speaking, an ethical will takes time to write, and even those of us who can get over the mortality issue find ourselves stuck on the simple logistical question: Where will I find the time? Because of this, I advise people to set aside only one hour to begin the process. We can all find one hour, and you'd be very surprised at how much you can write in an hour about what you believe in and what has been important to you that you'd like to pass down. If that is all you can give to the project, then an hour is more than nothing. But try to use that hour as a starting point and then schedule a few hours over the next weeks to add to the document. Put it into your calendar so that it appears as an appointment, an appointment with yourself.

And after it's written, you may also want to look at it and review it periodically. People make changes to their financial wills occasionally, so it is not surprising that people make changes to their ethical wills over time and with gained experience. They remember a piece of advice they got from a friend or relative that they would love to include, or they want to add what they learned from an experience they recently had. Once you complete your ethical will, it should be given to the estate lawyer or planner who is in possession of your financial will. I recommend having two copies so that you can add to the one you have and then turn in a revised document. You never know when it will be relevant so it is important that it is in a safe but accessible place.

Many ethical will counselors and services recommend writing an ethical will by hand, since your handwriting is one of the signature hallmarks of the self. People who inherit ethical wills often comment on the importance of the handwriting as yet another touchstone of authenticity and connection.

One reason to write an ethical will on a computer is so that you can revise or add to it with relative ease, since once you begin the process, it is common to think of more things to add over time. Another important reason is legibility: if you could have gone to medical school because your handwriting is *that* bad, it's probably a better idea to stick with a clear font on a computer. You don't want fights breaking out among your children because they can't read what you wrote. (I am reminded of the wonderful scene in Woody Allen's movie *Take the Money and Run*, where he hands a teller a note as he is trying to rob the bank and they argue about whether it says "I have a gun" or "I have a gub." It's best to avoid future second-guessing that you won't be around to clarify.)

Some people choose to make a film or a video as their ethical will, which has the added benefit of preserving the voice, another signature aspect of the self. The problem with this method as an exclusive way of leaving an ethical legacy is that technology changes so rapidly that people may not be able to access it some years in the future or may only access it at significant expense. If you captured your graduation on VHS or your first-dance wedding song on a cassette tape, you know exactly what I mean.

The letter remains the most effective format because it forces the writer to address the reader; it becomes more personal as a letter and less a rambling rumination on one's life. Someone specific is receiving the document, and that person or group will be in the writer's mind in a more deliberate way if it is a letter. This is important when thinking about length, tone and language. An ethical will is not a memoir or a life report.

When you can give advice that is in bullet points, it has greater staying power, and that's what you're after. The shorter the better. I recommend that, in letter form, the document be no more than ten pages long, and half that makes for even more compelling reading. It's less onerous to read and less onerous to write. In terms of minimizing the length, it may be helpful to make it as long as necessary in the initial writing and then shorten it once you've let everything spill out on paper. In the process, you want to be reading this out loud, imagining that you are a recipient. Don't hold back. If you can reduce it to one page, its impact may be even greater. Another option and a good way to get started is to write ten life principles or lessons you've learned or you live by.

There are many companies online that offer ethical will services, and if it helps motivate you to actually get it done, then by all means, pay for the assistance. But before you go that route, try your hand at writing down answers to the prompts below. The suggestions are grouped by theme to help you structure your final letter in coherent paragraphs. Some sections are much more emotionally charged than others. Try to do one section a sitting, so that the task does not feel so cumbersome that you quit.

In many ways, the term "ethical will" is not comprehensive enough to describe this document. It is really a life legacy that includes ethical advice but so much more: part memoir, part family history, part fiction. The recommended themes should help you organize your thoughts and pave the way to a meaningful goodbye. Think about answers and then condense them into a letter format.

## Personal Information

- Birthdate, birth place, information about your hometown
- Favorite photo of yourself and why
- Your personal story/history
- Transformative events in your life
- Historical events that you lived through that shaped the way you think and act
- Objects of significance that tell a piece of your life story. This may also be a way to give away objects of emotional significance rather than material worth. You may want to attach the object to a story and a blessing.

## Personal Happiness and Satisfaction

- Most impactful quote
- Places of significance to you and why
- Small things that have brought you happiness
- Favorite or important rituals
- Role of religion/spirituality in your life
- Favorite prayer

## The Role of Others

- Enumerating what you love about each person who is significant in your life
- Thanking and acknowledging what each significant person in your life has brought to you
- What you learned from your parents
- What your children taught you
- Thoughts on family

## Life Advice

- Your spiritual values or rules you live by
- Your life advice about friendship
- Your life advice about love/marriage
- Your life advice about work
- Your life advice about education/knowledge

## Finances

- Most important charitable causes and why
- How you used money to make a difference
- Your life advice about money

## Forgiveness

- Regrets
- Mistakes
- Request for forgiveness generally or from certain individuals
- Granting of forgiveness generally or to certain individuals

## Burial Requests

- Type of burial
- Location of burial
- Requested speakers at the funeral
- Requested rituals at the funeral, including prayer, poems and songs to be included

## Wishes for the Next Generation

- .................................................................................
- .................................................................................
- .................................................................................
- .................................................................................
- .................................................................................

## What You Will Miss Most

- .................................................................................
- .................................................................................
- .................................................................................
- .................................................................................
- .................................................................................

# Acknowledgments

Most authors acknowledge the people who helped them write a book. Many of my thank-you notes will never be read; I cannot thank the people who died before and during the writing of this book, but I will anyway. Please know that both in your lives and in your deaths you gave meaning to being human. I want to thank all the family and friends who spoke to me about traveling through the process of losing you and conferring greater meaning on life's only guaranteed experience through their relationship to you.

Some of those I interviewed proudly attached their names to their experiences. Others did so with hesitation. Some contributed only on condition of anonymity. I respect each decision. Consequently, many names and identifying details in this book have been masked to protect the dignity and memory of the dead and the living. Thank you for being brave enough to speak at all.

To Jon Karp, Nick Greene, and the wonderful team at Simon & Schuster: Publicists Andrea Rogoff and Meg Cassidy, Online Marketing Manager Elina Vaysbeyn, Assistant Managing Editor Gina DiMascia, Executive Managing Editor Irene Kheradi, Production Editor Loretta Denner, and Production Manager Michael Kwan: Thank you for taking the risk. You could not have been more gracious and loving with your edits and more inspirational with your commitment to this project. You have introduced so many lasting words to a world of flux and impermanence. May your wonderful books live beyond you.

To my students, my close friends and colleagues—I learn from you daily. A special shout-out to special friends: David Gregory, David Brooks, Jeffrey Goldberg, Steven Weisman, Daniel Silva, Frank Foer and Martin Indyk, who have made so much possible. To Sharon Mazel: friend, reader and editor. To the Avi Chai Foundation, the Covenant Foundation, the Mandel Foundation, and the Wexner Foundation, and to my friends at the Jewish Federation of Greater Washington: Thank you for years of support.

To my beloved grandmother, Celia, who—at 99—bewilders me with her strength and longevity. To my parents and extended family for showing me how to age gracefully. To my husband, Jeremy, and my four remarkable children—Talia, Gavriel, Yishai and Ayelet—may this be a small offering on the altar of mercy. Do not waste a moment in giving back to the world that has given you so much. You have given me so much. And to my Aunt Diane, to whom this book is dedicated. May God grant you the happiness you have always deserved for your overly generous heart.

Finally, I am most grateful to my Creator who has blessed me with this remarkable life.

# Notes

### Preface: Overcoming the Fear of Death

1. Michel de Montaigne, *The Essays of Michel de Montaigne*, trans. and ed. M. A. Screech (London: Allen Lane, 1991): 95.

### Chapter One: The Business of Death

1. E. Kay Trimberger, *The New Single Woman* (Boston: Beacon Press, 2005).
2. http://www.psychologytoday.com/blog/living-single/200901/the-ultimate -threat-single-people-youll-die-alone.
3. James L. Kugel, *In the Valley of the Shadow: On the Foundations of Religious Belief* (New York: Free Press, 2011): 3.
4. As seen in *The New Yorker* online (April 25, 2011): http://www.newyorker .com/reporting/2011/04/25/110425fa_fact_bilger.
5. Tom Jokinen, *Curtains: Adventures of an Undertaker-in-Training* (Philadelphia: Da Capo Press, 2010): 37.
6. Audrey Gordon, "The Psychological Wisdom of the Law," in *Jewish Reflections on Death*, ed. Jack Riemer (New York: Schocken Books, 1974): 98.
7. David Sipress cartoon, *The New Yorker* (July 4, 2011): 33.
8. Mary Roach, *Stiff: The Curious Lives of Human Cadavers* (New York: W.W. Norton, 2003): 82.
9. Jokinen, *Curtains*: 147.
10. Jessica Mitford, *The American Way of Death Revisited* (New York: Vintage, 2000): 7.
11. Bruce Feiler, "Mourning in a Digital Age," *New York Times* (January 15, 2012), Sunday Styles: 2.

12. Max Rivlin-Nadler, "*What Remains: Conversations with America's Funeral Directors.*" See http://www.theawl.com/2012/01/what-remains-conversations-with-americas-funeral-directors.

13. Jokinen, *Curtains*: 46.

14. Robert N. Bellah, Richard Madsen, William M. Sullivan, Ann Swidler, Steven M. Tipton, *Habits of the Heart: Individualism and Commitment in American Life* (Berkeley: University of California Press, 1996): 163.

15. David Eagleman, *Sum: Forty Tales from the Afterlives* (New York: Vintage, 2010): 23.

16. Feiler, "Mourning in a Digital Age": 2.

17. Bob Deits, *Life After Loss: A Practical Guide to Renewing Your Life after Experiencing Major Loss* (Philadelphia: Da Capo Press, 2009): 26.

18. Stephen Mitchell, ed., *The Selected Poetry of Rainer Maria Rilke* (New York: Vintage, 1989): 145

## Chapter Two: Pondering the Afterlife

1. Mark Twain, *Letters from the Earth* (Sioux Falls, SD: NuVision Publications, LLC, 2008): 15.

2. See Key Findings of "U.S. Religious Landscape Survey" at http://religions.pewforum.org/pdf/report2religious-landscape-study-key-findings.pdf.

3. As told to his friend Gehlek Rimpoche, who recorded it in *Good Life, Good Death: Tibetan Wisdom on Reincarnation* (New York: Riverhead Books, 2001): 151.

4. As seen in George Gallup and William Proctor, *Adventures in Immortality: A Look Beyond the Threshold of Death* (London: Souvenir, 1983).

5. Jeffrey Long, M.D., with Paul Perry, *Evidence of the Afterlife: The Science of Near-Death Experiences* (New York: HarperOne, 2010): 3.

6. Long, *Evidence of the Afterlife*: 6–7.

7. Long, *Evidence of the Afterlife*: 180.

8. See Kenneth Ring, *Heading Toward Omega: In Search of the Meaning of the Near-Death Experience* (New York: William Morrow, 1984).

9. From Dr. Leviton's *Washington Post Magazine* obituary, "A Professor of Death, and a Teacher to the End," by Emily Langer (December 15, 2011): 25.

10. Elisabeth Kübler-Ross, *On Death and Dying* (New York: Collier, 1993): 14.

11. Kübler-Ross, *On Death and Dying*: 14.

12. As quoted in Theodore Flournoy, *Spiritism and Psychology* (New York: Cosimo Classic, 2007): 52.

13. See article on Myers in *Encyclopedia of the Occult and Parapsychology*, by Lewis Spence (Whitefish, MT: Kessinger Publishing, LLC, 2003): 629.

14. See John Gray, *The Immortalization Commission: Science and the Strange Quest to Cheat Death* (New York: Farrar, Straus and Giroux, 2011).

15. Burkhard Bilger, "The Possibilian," in *The New Yorker* (April 25, 2011), as seen at http://www.newyorker.com/reporting/2011/04/25/110425fa_fact_bilger.

16. David Eagleman, *Sum: Forty Tales from the Afterlives* (New York: Vintage, 2010): 105–60.

17. As presented in Malcolm David Eckel, "Buddhism," The Great Courses, tape #3.

18. Rimpoche, *Good Life, Good Death*: ix.

19. Rimpoche, *Good Life, Good Death*: x.

20. In his foreword to Sogyal Rinpoche, *The Tibetan Book of Living and Dying* (New York: Harper One, 2002): ix.

21. Richard Gere, foreword to Matteo Pistono, *In the Shadow of the Buddha: Secret Journeys, Sacred Histories, and Spiritual Discovery in Tibet* (New York: Dutton, 2011): ix.

22. Rimpoche, *Good Life, Good Death*: 20–21.

## *Chapter Three: Sanctifying the Body in Death*

1. Sherwin B. Nuland, *How We Die* (New York: Knopf, 1994): 8.

2. Sogyal Rinpoche, *The Tibetan Book of Living and Dying* (New York: Harper One, 2002): 216.

3. Rinpoche, *Tibetan Book of Living and Dying*: 229.

4. Vivian Rakoff, "Psychiatric Aspects of Death in America," in *Death in American Experience*, ed. Arien Mack (New York: Schocken *Books*, 1973): 159.

5. Babylonian Talmud, *Shabbat*: 31a.

6. Ronna Kabatznick, "Preparing the Dead for Life's Final Passage," in Rochel U. Berman, *Dignity Beyond Death: The Jewish Preparation for Burial* (Jerusalem: Urim, 2005): 94.

7. Kabatznick, "Preparing the Dead": 95.

8. Irving Greenberg, foreword to Berman, *Dignity Beyond Death*: 13.

9. Jessica Mitford, *The American Way of Death Revisited* (New York: Vintage Books: 2000): 112.

10. Tom Jokinen, *Curtains: Adventures of an Undertaker-in-Training* (Philadelphia: Da Capo Press, 2010): 1.

11. Genesis 3:9.

12. Job 1:21.

13. Ecclesiastes 1:4, 8.

14. Job 14:7–10.

15. Hans Morgenthau, "Death in the Nuclear Age," in *Jewish Reflections on Death*, ed. Jack Riemer (New York: Schocken Books, 1974): 42.

16. Anton Chekhov, *Love and Other Stories* (Fairfield, IA: 1st World Library, 2006): 28.

17. To learn more, see http://whatisnaturalburial.org/

18. http://www.newschannel9.com/news/top-stories/stories/vid_519.shtml.

19. Jokinen, *Curtains*: 262.

20. Ecclesiastes Rabbah on Ecclesiastes 5:14.

## Chapter Four: Death as an Escape

1. Albert Camus, *The Myth of Sisyphus* (London: Vintage, 1991): 3.

2. Seneca, "Epistulae Morales," in *Letters from a Stoic*, trans. Robin Campbell (New York: Penguin Classics, 1969).

3. David Kuhl, M.D., *What Dying People Want: Practical Wisdom for the End of Life* (New York: Public Affairs, 2002): 22–23.

4. Kuhl, *What Dying People Want*: 22.

5. "Discworld's Terry Pratchett on Death and Deciding": http://www.npr .org/2011/08/11/139262401/discworlds-terry-pratchett-on-death-and-decid ing.

6. "Discworld's Terry Pratchett on Death and Deciding."

7. "Discworld's Terry Pratchett on Death and Deciding."

8. Sam Anderson, "'Twelve Polished Chapters Stacked Neatly on His Desk,'" *New York Times Magazine* (April 10, 2011): 52.

9. Dudley Clendinen, "The Good Short Life," in *New York Times*, Sunday Review (July 10, 2011): 4.

10. Clendinen, "The Good Short Life": 4.

11. David Brooks, "Death and Budgets" (July 14, 2011): http://www.nytimes .com/2011/07/15/opinion/15brooks.html?_r=1&hp.

12. C. G. Prado, *Coping with Choices to Die* (New York: Cambridge University Press: 2011): 20.

13. Prado, *Coping with Choices to Die*: 88–89.

14. Prado, *Coping with Choices to Die*: 88.

## Chapter Five: Denial, Resignation, Inspiration

1. See "Art Buchwald's Alive Again" (CBS News: Washington, Dec. 15, 2006).
2. Psalms 146:4.
3. Sherwin B. Nuland, *How We Die* (Knopf: New York, 1994): 224.
4. Nuland, *How We Die*: 258.
5. Nuland, *How We Die*: 244.
6. Nuland, *How We Die*: 244–45.
7. Elisabeth. Kübler-Ross, *On Death and Dying* (New York: Collier, 1993): 35.
8. Ernest Becker, *The Denial of Death* (New York: The Free Press, 1973): ix.
9. Psalms 55:5–6.
10. James C. Diggery and Doreen Z. Rothman, "Values Destroyed by Death," *Journal of Abnormal and Social Psychology* (vol. 63, issue 2), July 1961: 205–10.
11. Kübler-Ross, *On Death and Dying*: 2.
12. Psalms 89:49.
13. For the rest of his conclusions, see the column at: http://www.nytimes.com/2011/1½9/opinion/brooks-the-life-reports-ii.html?_r=1&emc=etal.
14. Bernard N. Schumacher, *Death and Mortality in Contemporary Philosophy* (New York: Cambridge University Press, 2011): 1.
15. Maggie Callanan, *Final Journeys: A Practical Guide for Bringing Care and Comfort at the End of Life* (New York: Bantam, 2009): 2–3.
16. Charles Krauthammer, "The Fine Art of Dying Well," in *Time* (March 5, 2007): http://www.time.com/time/magazine/article/0,9171,1595226,00.html.
17. Marilyn Webb, *The Good Death: The New American Search to Reshape the End of Life* (New York: Bantam Books, 1997): 1–27.

## Chapter Six: A Different Bucket List

1. Mitsuru Shimizu and Brett W. Pelham, "Postponing a Date with the Grim Reaper: Ceremonial Events and Mortality," in *Basic and Applied Social Psychology* (vol. 30, issue 1): 36–45.
2. José L. Wilches-Gutiérrez, Luz Arenas-Monreal, Alfredo Paulo-Maya, Ingris Peláez-Ballestas, Alvaro J. Idrovo, "A 'beautiful death': Mortality, death, and holidays in a Mexican municipality," in *Social Science & Medicine* (vol. 74, issue 5): 775–82.
3. See http://www.fresnobee.com/2011/02/22/2281160/friends-cant-face-woman-dying.html.

4. "Ask Amy," *Washington Post*, March 20, 2011, Local Living section: 19.

5. "Ask Amy," *Washington Post*.

6. Elisabeth Kübler-Ross, *On Life After Death* (Berkeley, CA: Celestial Arts, 2008): viii.

7. Ira Byock, *Dying Well: Peace and Possibilities at the End of Life* (New York: Riverhead Books, 1997): 53.

8. Byock, *Dying Well*: 25–26.

9. D. Spiegel, J.R. Bloom, H. Kramer, and E. Gottheil, Psychological support for cancer patients," *Lancet*, 1989 Dec 16:2 (8677):1447; F.I. Fawzy, N.W. Fawzy, et al., "Malignant melanoma. Effects of an early structured psychiatric intervention, coping, and affective state on recurrence and survival 6 years later," *Arch Gen Psychiatry* 1993 Sept: 50 (9): 681–89.

10. D. W. Kissane, A. Love, A. Hatton, et al., "Effect of Cognitive-Existential Group Therapy on Survival in Early-Stage Breast Cancer," in *Journal of Clinical Oncology* 2004 Nov 1: 22(21):4255–60. Published online on September 27, 2004. P. J. Goodwin, "Support Groups in Breast Cancer: When a Negative Result Is Positive," in *Journal of Clinical Oncology* 2004 Nov 1:22(21): 4244–46. Published online on September 27, 2004.

11. Maggie Callanan, *Final Journeys: A Practical Guide for Bringing Care and Comfort at the End of Life* (New York: Bantam, 2009): 18.

12. David Kessler, *The Needs of the Dying: A Guide for Bringing Hope, Comfort, and Love to Life's Final Chapter* (New York: HarperCollins, 1997): 2.

13. Kessler, *The Needs of the Dying*: 29.

14. David Kuhl, M.D.,*What Dying People Want: Practical Wisdom for the End of Life* (New York: Public Affairs, 2002): 52.

15. Byock, *Dying Well*: 32.

16. G. Leigh Wilkerson, RN, *Considering Comfort Care: A Guide for Families* (Fayetteville, AK: Limbertwig Press, 2008): 6.

17. Wilkerson, *Considering Comfort Care*: 28.

18. Mary Callaway and Frank D. Ferris, eds., "Advancing Palliative Care: The Public Health Perspective," *Journal of Pain and Symptom Management*, vol. 33, issue 5 (2007): 483–654; and Stephen R. Connor, Bruce Pyenson, Kathryn Fitch, Carol Spence, and Kosuke Iwasaki, "Comparing Hospice and Nonhospice Patient Survival Among Patients Who Die Within a Three-Year Window," vol. 33, issue 3 (March 2007): 238–46.

## Chapter Seven: Closing Words

1. From "The Lives They Loved," in *New York Times Magazine* (December 25, 2011): 50; and his granddaughter's reminiscences, http://paigegreen .wordpress.com/2011/09/26/you-made-my-life/.

2. Marianne Williamson, *A Return to Love* (New York: HarperCollins, 1992): 209–16.

3. Marilyn Johnson, *The Dead Beat: Lost Souls, Lucky Stiffs, and the Perverse Pleasures of Obituaries* (New York: HarperCollins, 2007): 9.

4. Johnson, *The Dead Beat*: 9–10.

5. Johnson, *The Dead Beat*: 117.

6. See http://www.obitwriters.org/awards2008.html (May 5, 2011).

7. Johnson, *The Dead Beat*: 37.

8. Jo Myers, *Good to Go: A Guide to Preparing for the End of Life* (New York: Sterling Publishing, 2010): 20.

9. Genesis 25:6.

10. Sogyal Rinpoche, *The Tibetan Book of Living and Dying* (New York: Harper One, 2002): 228.

11. Rimpoche Nawang Gehlek, *Good Life, Good Death: Tibetan Wisdom on Reincarnation* (New York: Riverhead Books, 2001): 154–55.

12. Rimpoche, *Good Life, Good Death*: 164.

13. Ecclesiastes 2: 18–22.

14. See John chapters 5–18.

15. Rashi and the *Sifrei* on Deuteronomy 1:1.

16. Jack Riemer and Nathaniel Stampfer, *Ethical Wills: A Modern Jewish Treasury* (New York: Schocken Books, 1983): xix.

17. Riemer and Stampfer, *Ethical Wills*: xx.

## Chapter Eight: The Last Apology

1. http://people-press.org/2006/01/05/strong-public-support-for-right-to-die/.

2. *Shulkhan Arukh* 338, as translated by Chaim N. Denburg, in "From the *Shulkhan Arukh*" in *Jewish Reflections on Death*, ed. Jack Riemer (New York: Schocken Books, 1974): 18.

3. See "Forgiveness and Justice: A Research Agenda for Social and Personality Psychology," by Julie Exline, Everett L. Worthington Jr., Peter Hill and

Michael E. McCullough, in *Personality and Social Psychology Review*, http://psr.sagepub.com/content/7/4/337.short for a study of the relationship between forgiveness and anger in a sample adult population in Taiwan.

4. Martin Luther King Jr., cited without attribution, in Johann Christoph Arnold, *Why Forgive?* (Farmington, PA: Plough Publishing House, 2000): 29.

5. Harriet Lerner, *The Dance of Connection: How to Talk to Someone When You're Mad, Hurt, Scared, Frustrated, Insulted, Betrayed, or Desperate* (New York: Harper, 2002): 5.

6. Simon Wiesenthal, *The Sunflower: On the Possibilities and Limits of Forgiveness* (New York: Schocken Books, 1976): 57.

7. Cynthia Ozick, in Wiesenthal, *The Sunflower*: 187.

8. Ira Byock, *Dying Well: Peace and Possibilities at the End of Life* (New York: Riverhead Books, 1997): 252–53.

9. As cited without attribution by David Kuhl, M.D., *What Dying People Want: Practical Wisdom for the End of Life* (New York: Public Affairs, 2002): 180–81.

10. See "Forgiveness by God, forgiveness of others and psychological well-being in late life," by Neal Krause and Christopher G. Ellison, in *Journal for the Scientific Study of Religion* http://onlinelibrary.wiley.com/doi/10.1111/1468 5906.00162/abstract.

11. Arnold, *Why Forgive?*: 30.

12. http://www.guardian.co.uk/uk/2008/oct/06/7.

## Chapter Nine: Learning from Grief

1. Philip Larkin, *Collected Poems*, ed. Anthony Thwaite (New York: Noonday Press, 1993): 298. I am grateful to Noam Osband who reminded me just how remarkably Larkin captures the heartbreak of grief.

2. The literature on this subject is complex and controversial, with some of the studies criticized as poor examples of medical research. See K. Masters, G. Spielmans, J. Goodson, "Are there demonstrable effects of distant intercessory prayer? A meta-analytic review" in *Annals of Behavioral Medicine* 2006 Aug: 32(1): 21–26; David R. Hodge, "A Systematic Review of the Empirical Literature on Intercessory Prayer," in *Research on Social Work Practice* (March 2007) vol. 17 no. 2, 174–87 doi: 10.1177/1049731506296170; R. C. Byrd (July 1988), "Positive therapeutic effects of intercessory prayer in a coronary care unit population,"in *Southern Medical Journal* 81 (7): 826–29. For a contrasting view, see H. Benson, J. A. Dusek, J. B. Sherwood, P. Lam, C. F. Bethea, W. Carpenter, S. Levitsky, P. C. Hill, D. W. Clem Jr.,

M. K. Jain, D. Drumel, S. L. Kopecky, P. S. Mueller, D. Marek, S. Rollins, and P. L. Hibbard. "Study of the Therapeutic Effects of Intercessory Prayer (STEP) in cardiac bypass patients: a multicenter randomized trial of uncertainty and certainty of receiving intercessory prayer," http://www.ncbi.nlm.nih.gov/pubmed/16569567.

3. Maggie Callanan, *Final Journeys: A Practical Guide for Bringing Care and Comfort at the End of Life* (New York: Bantam, 2009):120.

4. Song of Songs 8:6.

5. Plutarch, *The Lives of Noble Grecians and Romans* (New York: Modern Library, n.d.): 110; N. Lewis and M. Reinhold, *Roman Civilization* (New York: Columbia University Press, 1959): 1108, as seen in *The JPS Torah Commentary*, ed. Jeffrey H. Tigay (Philadelphia: The Jewish Publication Society, 1996): 136.

6. Deuteronomy 14:1.

7. Samson Raphael Hirsch, commentary on the Pentateuch, Deuteronomy 14:1 (Gateshead, England: Judaic Press, 1976): 242.

8. Hirsch, commentary on the Pentateuch.

9. Callanan, *Final Journeys*: 109.

10. Joseph B. Soloveitchik, "The Halakhah of the First Day," in *Jewish Reflections on Death*, ed. Jack Riemer (New York: Schocken Books, 1974): 76.

11. Soloveitchik, "The Halakhah of the First Day": 79.

12. *Shulkhan Arukh* (lit. "The Set Table"): #394, laws 1 and 6.

13. See Margaret Stroebe, Henk Schut, and Wolfgang Stroebe, "Attachment in Coping With Bereavement: A Theoretical Integration" in *Review of General Psychology*, vol. 9 (1), Mar 2005: 48–66.

14. As seen in Perry Garfinkel, "Men in Grief Seek Others Who Mourn as They Do," in *New York Times* (July 26, 2011): D-5.

15. Garfinkel, "Men in Grief."

16. C. S. Lewis, *A Grief Observed* (New York: Harper, 1996): 18–19. With special thanks to Meir for my copy.

17. Greenberg in *Dignity Beyond Death*: 12.

18. Lewis, *A Grief Observed*: 9–10.

19. Lewis, *A Grief Observed*: 33.

20. Lewis, *A Grief Observed*: 53.

21. Richard Neuhaus, *As I Lay Dying: Meditations Upon Returning* (New York: Basic Books, 2003): 161.

22. Lewis, *A Grief Observed*: 25.

## Chapter Ten: Using Death to Change Your Life

1. Job 28: 20–22.

2. Babylonian Talmud, *Brakhot* 30b.

3. A. J. Heschel, *Moral Grandeur and Spiritual Audacity* (New York: Farrar, Straus and Giroux, 1997): 366.

4. Sherwin B. Nuland, How We Die (New York: Knopf, 1994): xvi.

5. Babylonian Talmud *Eruvin* 13b.

6. Jean Paul Sartre, *Being and Nothingness: An Essay in Phenomenological Ontology* (Secaucus, NJ: Citadel Press, 2001): 515.

7. Epicurus, "Letter to Menoeceus," in *Letter Writing in Greco-Roman Antiquity*, ed. Stanley Kent Stowers (Louisville, KY: Westminster John Knox Press, 1986) :117.

8. Epicurus, 35.

9. Bernard N. Schumacher, *Death and Mortality in Contemporary Philosophy* (New York: Cambridge University Press, 2011): 124.

10. Psalm 14:1.

# About the Author

Dr. Erica Brown is a writer and educator who lives in the D.C. area with her husband, four children and two dogs.